A Guide to Medical Teaching and Learning Training of the Trainers (TOT)

In the View of the Learner-Centered Learning Model

Dr. Abdullah Dukhail Al-Khatami

ISBN
978-1-5437-4596-2 (sc)
978-1-5437-45979 (e)

Print information available on the last page.

To order additional copies of this book, contact
Toll Free 800 101 2657 (Singapore)
Toll Free 1 800 81 7340 (Malaysia)
www.partridgepublishing.com/singapore
orders.singapore@partridgepublishing.com

07/25/2018

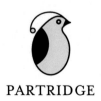

PARTRIDGE

A Guide to Medical Teaching & Learning

Training of the Trainers (TOT)

In the view of the

Learner-centered Learning Model

By Dr. Abdullah Dukhail Al-Khatami

CONTRIBUTERS:

1. Dr.Nada A. Albunaian

Family Medicine Consultant
Master of Health Professional Education- Maastricht University Holland
Trainer in SPFM program in MOH-Eastern province, Saudi Arabia

2. Dr. Abdulaillah ALQurashi

Family Medicine Consultant
Master of Medical Education
Trainer in Saudi board of Family Medicine in National Guard Jeddah, Saudi Arabia

3. Dr. Shatha Al Zuhair

Family Medicine Consultant
Trainer in SPFM program in MOH-Eastern province, Saudi Arabia

Acknowledgment

Perseverance is an attribute that allows anyone to accomplish a daunting task in life. I am full of gratitude to Almighty Allah for bestowing me such an attribute; it ameliorated in transcribing the ideas into the publishable artifact.

A lot of inspiration for these ideas are the contributions of many individuals whom I came across while playing different roles in my life. I would like to extend my gratitude to all these individuals (facilitators & learners). Especially the participants who attended the "training of the trainers" courses and enriched the ideas.

Hats off to The Royal College of Physicians and Surgeons of Canada for promulgation of CanMEDs, a widely accepted and applied physician competency framework in the contemporary world.
Finally, a bundle of thanks to my family for enhanced caring and sharing attitude during intellectual infatuation for this project

Preface:

Medical education is continually changing, as the health care needs of our populations change and as new knowledge emerges about the best ways to prepare future clinicians.

In this new book, Abdullah Al-Khathami, Family and Community Medicine consultant, senior medical educator and global leader in primary care mental health, outlines his ideas about refocusing medical education to become more centred on meeting the specific learning needs of our future doctors.

A century after Flexner, and 50 years after the development of problem-based learning approaches, our medical education is ready to be transformed once again, to ensure that our medical graduates are equipped to meet the health care challenges of the 21st century. Our medical education needs to embrace true person-centred care. Our medical education needs to adapt to new technology, both used by clinicians and by the people we serve. Our medical education needs to be incorporated into our daily work, so that we learn while we work, and have our daily activity presented back to us for reflection, and new technology and clinical decision support provides the capacity to do this. Our medical education needs a global perspective, as many of our graduates will work all around the world. Our medical education needs to acknowledge the social determinants of health and respect diversity and human rights. Our medical education needs to be based on ensuring safe, high quality and appropriate health care made available to all people.

This book helps us to reshape the training we provide to our future doctors and to ensure that we centre our teaching on their future professional needs. Through nine chapters, Dr Al-Khathami leads the reader through some of the latest thinking on effective teaching and learning skills, assisting teachers to develop their planning and presentation skills based on the clinical contexts where our future doctors will work. The book refocuses our approaches to supervision and work-based assessment, and concludes with the practical application of the desired roles and abilities our future doctors will require if they are to effectively meet the health care needs of the people they serve.

If you are a medical teacher, or a medical learner, you will find this book supports your effectiveness both as teacher and learner, while enhancing both your professional development and your future work as a confident and competent clinician.

Professor Michael Kidd

Chair, Department of Family Medicine, University of Toronto, Canada (2017-)

Professorial Fellow, Murdoch Children's Research Institute, Australia (2017-)

Dean, Faculty of Medicine, Nursing and Health Sciences, Flinders University, Australia (2009-2016)

Chair, Department of General Practice, The University of Sydney, Australia (1996-2008)

President, World Organization of Family Doctors (2013-2016)

President, Royal Australian College of General Practitioners (2002-2006)

Introduction

The world is witnessing a paradigm shift from teacher led to learner-centered model. This driver of change has posed new demands on all, (and especially) the key stakeholders (Trainers, Trainees/Learners). This book is an endeavor to facilitate the key stakeholders of medical specialties in conceptualizing the modern concepts and utilizing the techniques and methods for learner-centered learning. In order to extend the scope of the target audience, the adopted structure and style is kept simple and general, so that non-medical audience can also get benefit from it.

After fifteen of teaching trainers in different specialties, publishing this book has evolved to give you an easy-to-use modern concept, techniques, and methods to teach others or to learn based on the concept of the "Learner-Central Learning Model". Looking to preserve the learning and training only in the time of activities without home-tasks.

This book consists of 9 chapters. The chapters one to four are providing the knowledge and the skills needed for the teachers and learners in the classrooms to achieve the required learning materials. The chapters from five to seven are providing the knowledge and the skills required for the teachers and learners in the clinical settings to achieve the required learning subjects. Chapter eight discuss the purpose of the supervision meeting between the learners and their supervisors, office learning. The last chapter is discussing the CanMEDs roles and how to apply and assess them in the medical learning environment in a concise and well-structured way.

Chapter one "effective teaching and learning skills." It looks at the importance of an understanding of this model as a modern learning model to replace the traditional model, teacher-center model which depend on a lecture as a method of teaching and learning. It covers trainer's competencies, learner-centered learning (LCL) model, learning skills (metacognition), facilitator's skills, learner motivation, and feedback and reflection.

Chapter two "small-group teaching and learning methods." It discusses the reasons for teaching in small groups, small-group teaching techniques, and methods (10 types), the tutor roles in small-group teaching.

Chapter three "Teaching and Planning", one of the most critical roles of the teacher is planning. Proper planning provides a structure and context for both teacher and learner. It sets out the importance of teaching planning, individual sessions, course planning, the requirements of preparation, and the planning framework.

Chapter-four "presentation skills," the presentation is a type of communication between the teachers and their students in which, it should be attractive, and help for clarifying the subject.

Chapter- five "clinical teaching skills", the clinical teaching is at the core of teaching and learning in medicine, involving patients, their problems, and their illnesses. It is a demanding task. The teachers are provided by teaching skills for both juniors and senior learners in a busy clinics. It is feedback and reflection based learning.

Chapter six "5-micro-skills for clinical teaching" (the one-minute preceptor). It is suitable for senior learners rather juniors in the context of busy clinical practice. Applying 5-micro-skills enables the preceptor to be an efficient assessor, instructor, and feedback provider.

Chapter seven "work-based assessment." It based on a formative assessment and constructive feedback. In this chapter focuses on three common assessment methods; mini CEX, DOPS, and CBD.

Chapter eight "academic supervision meetings and portfolio assessment." It clarifies the portfolio types, with emphasis on the selection/task portfolio. Different between the teacher role in a clinic and the supervision meeting in the office.

Chapter nine "CanMEDS Roles in Medical Practice" it was developed by the Canadian Royal College in 1996 as a framework for improving patient care by enhancing physician training. Here, I tried the best to make them easy applied in our clinics, and how to practice and assess each role in a teaching environment.

Hopefully, this book helps both trainers and learners to enhance their knowledge and skills, improve their practice efficiently and effectively, promote the clinical independence, prepare learners for optimal health care for their patients, and become a competent, independent, and collaborative clinicians who able to be efficient in the time-management. All these achievements will be in a "No home-task training."

Dr. Abdullah D. Al-Khathami

Contents

List of abbreviation

a.m.	ante meridiem
ASSURE	(Analyze Learners, State Standards and Objectives, Select Strategies, Technology, Media, and Materials, Utilize Technology, Media, and Materials, Require Learner Participation, Evaluate and Revise
BPE	Blinded Patient Encounters
CanMEDS	Canadian Medical Education Directives for Specialists
CBD	Case-Based Discussion
CEC	Clinical Encounter Cards
CWS	Clinical Work Sampling
DOPS	Direct Observation of Procedural Skills
Dr	Doctor
DVD	Digital Video Disc
e.g	exempli gratia
HDR	Half Day Release
ICE	Idea, Concern, Expectation
IV	Intravenous
LCL	Learner-Centred Learning
MCQ	Multiple Choice Question
Mg	Micrograms
mini CEX	mini Clinical Evaluation Exercise
MOH	Ministry Of Health
MSF	Multi-Source Feedback
OSCE	Objective Structured Clinical Examination
p.m	post meridiem
SBFM	Saudi Board Family Medicine
TOT	Training of Trainers
WBA	Work-Based Assessment
Wks	Weeks

List of illustration

List of tables

Chapter 1

Effective Teaching and Learning Skills

1. EFFECTIVE TEACHING AND LEARNING SKILLS

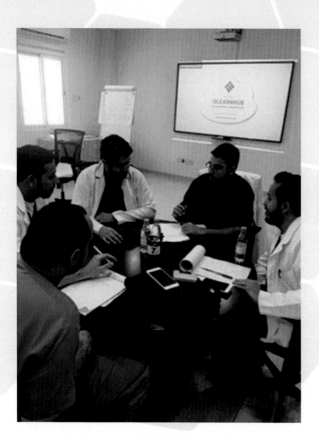

This chapter looks at the importance of understanding learning needs and applying the best teaching and learning methods to meet these needs.

It helps teachers and learners to choose the appropriate learning methods and develop the best approaches to ensure a high level of learning achievement results.

Overview of Chapter 1

- Trainer's competencies
- Learner-centred learning (LCL) model
- Learning skills (metacognition)
- Facilitator's skills
- Learner motivation
- Feedback and reflection

1.1 TRAINER'S COMPETENCIES

The Latin verb docere, or "to teach", is at the root of being a doctor. There are three roles for staff in academic medicine.

I. Clinical care
II. Research
III. Teaching

Good teaching requires skills that must be learned.

It is universally agreed that teachers should be trained formally in basic education methods.

The goal of teachers should not be excellence in teaching but, rather, an excellence in ensuring that their students are good learners (Amin and Eng, 2006).

Minimum Competency of Medical Teachers

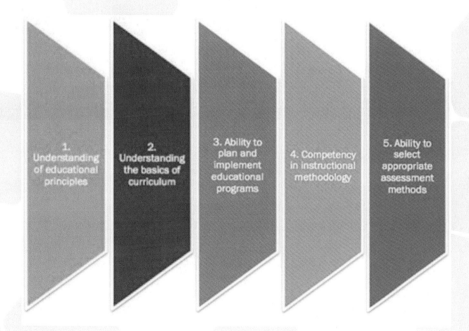

1. Understanding of Educational Principles

2. Understanding the basics of Curriculum

3. Ability to plan & implement Educational Program

4. Competency in Instructional Methodology rang

5. Ability to choose proper Assessment Methods

- Educational Principles

Understanding learning theories leads to

- Familiarity of terminology frequently used in medical education literature.
- Underpinning educational practice by educational principles.
- Recognizing the ineffectiveness of educational practice without theoretical construction.
- Conceptualizing students as learners and teachers as facilitators among "adult learners" and in the field of "andragogy".
- Developing skills of learning (metacognition) as the most effective and efficient way to achieve learning.

Medical education has been transformed by several influential theories of learning.

- Learner-centred learning, for example, cognitive theory, constructive theory
- Experimental learning, for example, behaviorism
- Self-directed learning, for example, constructive theory

- Curriculum and Educational Programs

New educational programs are built on a modified curriculum utilizing the concept of the LCL model. This model attains adult-learning principles through applying a modern instructional methodology. Various small-group learning and teaching techniques and methods, in the presence of a competent teacher, can attain the concept of the LCL model.

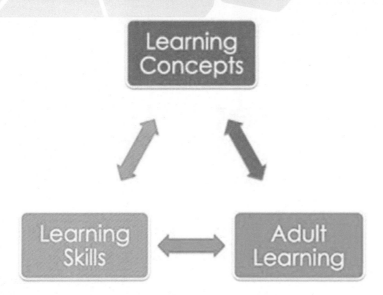

- Instructional Methodology

Medical education works to improve instructional methods through

- Shifting traditional methods, adapting lectures to be more interactive, using small-group learning to achieve particular needs and goals—a 'learner-centred approach.'
- Establishing new curricula and training strategies based on the learner-centred approach; for example, case-based learning moves the learning process to be more effective and efficient.

Applying modern instructional methodology needs a medical teacher who

1. Understands the core principles and educational rationale of the LCL model

2. Understands various options of teaching methods or learning achievements, particularly the efficient methods

3. Masters the various effective facilitator skills

Is able to assess the learners' learning achievements

- Innovation in Clinical Teaching Methodology

Improvement in instructional methods is not limited to classroom teaching. It also involves clinical education, shifting from traditional disease-based teaching to a patient-centred approach and "person-centred care. Modern techniques and methods have been implemented towards conducting effective clinical teaching.

Clinical competencies—such as appropriate communication skills, patient-central interview approach, selectivity, clinical reasoning, and professionalism—were structured in the clinical teaching.

Innovation models, considering the learners' needs and levels—such as five microskill steps for clinical teaching, reflection, and constructive feedback—have been implemented for delivering clinical teaching.

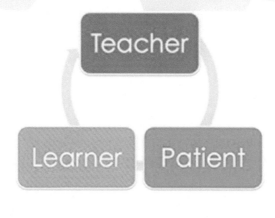

New learning approach

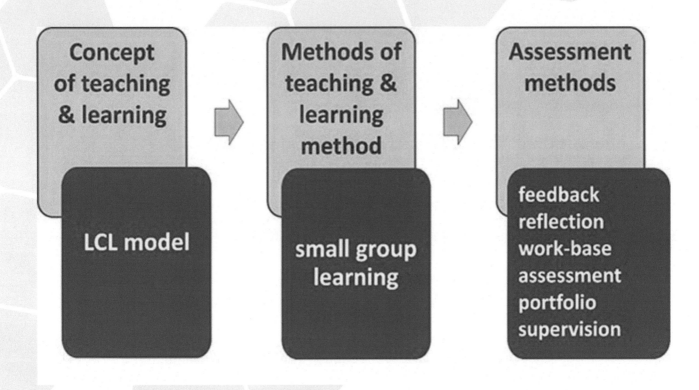

Competency Domains in Family Medicine Practice

There are four major domains.

1. Skills Dimension of Competencies in Clinical Practice
(College of Family Physicians of Canada, 2010, explained in the medical clinical competencies Chpter-5)

> 1. Appropriate communication skills
> 2. Patient-centeredness
> 3. Professionalism
> 4. Selectivity
> 5. Clinical reasoning skills
> 6. Procedure skills

2. Phases of the Clinical Encounter

The clinical encounters have a primary function in the cognitive process assessment guidance that mostly relies on a particular decision based on an accurate presentation. It includes the clinical solving and decision-making skills that undergo a hypothetical or constructive process.

3. Priority Topics, Core Procedures, and Themes

These constitute a list of problems or situations the competent physician should be able to do in independent practice.

Priority Topics: Includes diagnose, management, as well as related roles e.g. discovering the hidden agenda or the real problem, periodic health screening, education and promotion task. All these depend how physician competent in the "Selectivity competency".

Core Procedures: Mastering the needed technical skills required for core procedures.

Themes: Its complex of combining different competencies or skills: communication skills, patient-centred approach, professionalism, and clinical reasoning.

4. Key Features and Observable Behaviors

Observation, peer review, or recording assessments are operational evaluations describing the ability to apply clinical competencies in daily clinical work.

Teaching and Patient Care

In improving teaching and learning methods based on educational theories and derived principles, such as the LCL model, the gap between educational theory and practice can be filled by the LCL. Consequently, medical educators will be competent teachers and able to improve the next generation of teachers. As a result, they will provide a higher level of patient care and improve outcomes.

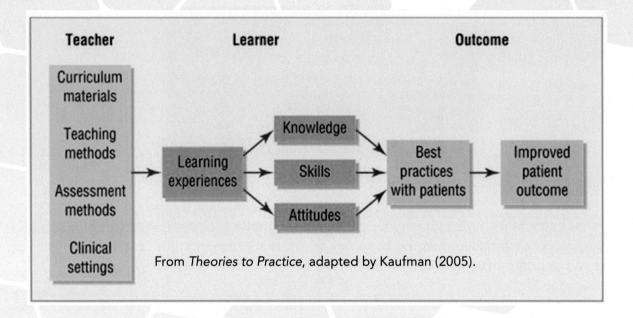

From *Theories to Practice*, adapted by Kaufman (2005).

1.2 LEARNER-CENTRED LEARNING

This section focuses on the LCL model for the learning and teaching processes and exploring.

- How we identify what our current educational status is, and where it should be.
- The barriers to implementing LCL.
- How we promote training centres in the context of LCL.

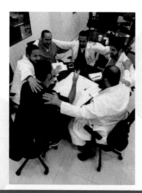

- Definitions

The teacher-centered approach is known as a traditional instructional approach. Teacher try to deliver a massage to the learners without ensuring the massage is achieved or not, the learners responsible to look after that.

The LCL model is considered a modern approach in which the learner is actively and effectively engaged in the learning process to master a particular task and create a positive attitude towards it (Ahmad and Aziz, 2009).

In a learner-centered class, learners participate in leading discussions, and teachers become facilitators. The teacher's role is to facilitate the learners' discussion, allowing learners to learn, use, and explore the learning materials (Eken, 2000; Ahmad and Aziz, 2009).

Facilitators guides the discussion towards achieving the aim of the session, highlight the main points, helps to define the learning gap, and able to assess the learning achievement.

LCL Rationale

It is estimated that medical knowledge doubles every five years. What is being taught in medical school loses its relevance during working years (Amin and Eng, 2006).

LCL shifts the instructor's role from information provider to a facilitator of the learning process.

The last decade has seen

- A new vision for learning developed by the Association of American Colleges and Universities (2002). There has been much discussion about learner-centred teaching as a new model for teaching and learning.

   The LCL model recognizes there is no unified theory to explain every aspect of learning.

Also, with progressive education in the nineteenth century and the influence of psychologists, the way in which learners determine or share their needs determines the way they are taught and what they are taught. Some educators have largely replaced traditional curriculum approaches with "group work".

Cooperative learning (learner-centered) applies an effective and efficient learning approach, resulting in a significantly higher mean achievement score compared to the regular teaching (teacher-centered) approach (Muraya and Kimano, 2011).

Learning Complexity

Cognitive Domain (Bloom's Taxonomy,, 1956)

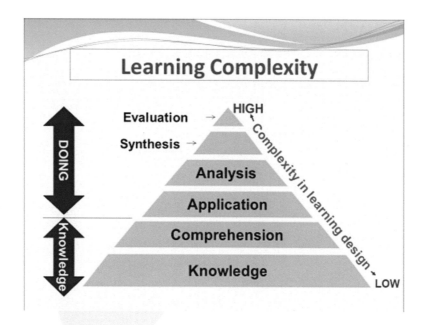

Knowledge: remembering previously learned material

    Examples of related verbs: identify, list, record, recognize, acquire

    Skills you learn: recall, memorize

Comprehension/Understanding: ability to construct meaning from material

    Examples of related verbs: report, recognize, explain, express, discuss, describe, review, differentiate

    Skills you learn: making conclusions, interpreting, summarizing, comparing

Application: ability to implement learned material in concrete situations

    Examples of related verbs: apply, develop, translate, use, operate, organize, employ, restructure, interpret, demonstrate, illustrate

    Skills you learn: practice, simulation

Analysis: breakdown of the material into its components so that its organizational structure may be better understood

    Examples of related verbs: analyse, compare, probe, inquire, examine, categorize, investigate, detect, classify

    Skills you learn: discovery, inspection, discrimination

Synthesis: combination of components or elements to form a connected whole

> *Examples of related verbs:* compose, produce, design, assemble, create, prepare, predict, modify, tell, set up, organize

> *Skills you learn:* planning, formulating, proposing, developing, arranging

Evaluation: ability to judge, check, critique the value of material

> *Examples of related verbs:* judge, assess, compare, evaluate, conclude, measure, estimate, argue, decide, choose

> *Skills you learn:* validation, appraisal, criticism

Training Methods and Learning Achievement percentage from the Conducting Session (Motorola University, 1996)

The Learners' achievement from:

- Lecture 5%
- Reading 10%
- Audiovisual 20%
- Demonstration 30%
- Group discussion 50%
- Practice by doing 75%
- Teaching others 90%

In teaching, it is not always necessary to prepare a session and teach others, which is the best. It also occurs when a group discusses an issue, and it is presented by one or more group members. Who presents the group answer is the one who achieves 90 per cent.

Teaching Approaches

Where Are We in Our Education?

	Traditional Approach	Modern Approach
Concept	Teaching	Learning
Approach/model	Teacher dominated	Learner-Centred Learning (LCL)
Process	Didactic/lectures	Small-group learning
Assessment concept	Summative exam	Formative and summative
Assessment tools	MCQ, OSCE, essay	Feedback and reflection, assessment forms, portfolios

- **Traditional learning**: focusses on superficial learning or memorization. LCL leads to deep learning, connecting current learning to learner experiences and enabling learners to organize their information.

- New Approach, LCL model: uses small-group learning as the learning process. Feedback, reflection, and work-based assessments measure the learning achievements.

Learner-Centred Teaching Dimensions

In shifting teaching to the LCL model, five practices need to be changed (Weimer, M, 2002).

1. Content function
   Learners need to understand and be actively engaged with their learning materials.

2. Instructor role
   a. Help student to learn.
   b. Create a safe learning environment.
   c. Adopt teaching methods appropriate for the learning goals.

3. Learning responsibility
   a. Shifts from the teachers to the learners.
   b. Instructors guide and motivate learners to become self-directed, lifelong learners.

4. Assessment processes purpose:
   a. Shifting from only assigning grades to include constructive feedback for the purpose of learning improvement.
   b. LCL model integrates assessment with feedback as part of the learning process.

5. Power balance: Teachers share some decision with learners

LCL and Self-efficacy (high achievement and grades)

Personal involvement: learner's needs, involve in a small group discussion…leads to:

Intrinsic motivation …. leads to personal commitment…..leads to high learning achievement…. leads for enhancing mastering competencies and ability to succeed …. Leads to self-efficacy that leads to high grads achieve.

LCL Model encourages self-reflection

LCL Model Advantages

- Prepares learners to be independent and self-reliant in their learning
- More responsive to fast changing needs
- Places emphasis on the learning process as well as content
- Effective and efficient
- Not only be effective; the capability of producing the desired result. LCL model is utilizing efficient learning methods which safe time and efforts.
- Leads into a deep learning: Focus on what mean, related new information to what already known and had experienced, work to organize and structure content, and see reading as important source of reading.

- Where the traditional learning leads into a superficial learning: Memorize fact, focus on elements of reading, failed to differentiate between evidence and information – Unreflective, and the task as external imposition (burden)
- LCL Model Features:
- Learner plays a more active and self-directed role
- Enhances learning by enabling self-reflection
- Offers an opportunity for the learners to identify their needs
- Encourages the intrinsic motivation for learning.
- Positions the teacher as a facilitator rather than a knowledge provider
- Learning methods bring together:
  a. Individual; through self-learning
  b. Social interaction; through small groups learning for exchange knowledge and learning experiences.
  c. Collaboration; between learners and facilitator to identify the learning gap, choose an efficient learning method, and assess the achievement with consulting and follow-up.

- Learning in the LCL Model is a shared activity between teacher and learners to determine:
  a. their own goals
  b. learning methods to achieve the goals
  c. learning process assessment

- Learning skills are required to enhance the learning achievement.

Application LCL Model Example:

During a medicine rotation, a 44-year old diabetic patient is admitted to the ward.

Whenever the doctor touches the patient's abdomen for examination, the patient vomits.

I asked why the patient vomits when his abdomen is touched. Our trainer threw the question back at, highlighting that I had made a good observation, but asking me to identify the answer and report back to him.

I was, indeed interested to find out the reason and felt very motivated to explore and discuss this together with my teacher.

After exploring different possible diagnosis, I found that hyponatremia was the cause. Hyponatremia causes muscular irritant of tough Abdomen muscles, leading to contractions which compress the diaphragm, resulting in vomiting when the stomach is touched. Also, hyponatremia is often found in diabetic patients.

Once I had collected this evidence, I shared my thinking with my trainer; he listened, and then said: "That is great- well done!"

The patient's condition and my diagnosis has stuck in my memory ever since.

Had my teacher simply answered by initial question, I could have forgotten the information a few years later- simply because I had not involved in the process of finding out the knowledge.

TASK:

Find evidence from this story which reflects each Learner-Central Learning features

Barriers to Implementing LCL Model

Teacher's Viewpoints:

Personal issue, change resistant

Haven't the collaborative work skills

They don't have the skills needed for the new approach

Learner's Viewpoints

- Learners may feel vulnerable and reluctant to join group discussions if they are not sufficiently trained in learner skills
- Learners need to understand how LCL works
- Learners may have difficulty assessing LCL, as it is a high-order cognitive process

Teacher Roles in LCL model

- Should be less directive and more facilitative.
- Help learners to define their goals based on their needs.
- Emphasis on the learning process as well as the content.
- Teach principles with wider appeals and applications, not esotericism.
- Introduce variations of learning methods, e.g. different types of small groups learning
- Make lecture, when it is necessary, interactive.
- The lecture should not be the primary teaching method.
- The teacher should encourage:
  - A. Case-based teaching
  - B. Small groups discussion
  - C. Peer review
  - D. Promote self-reflection and self-assessment
- How learning skills can be inspired among our trainees

1.3 Learning Skills (Metacognition)

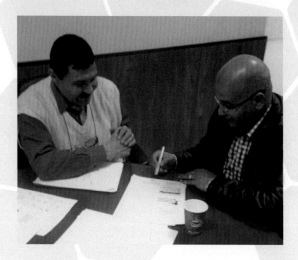

This section looks at:

- Concepts of learning skills
- Essential skills needed to apply LCL

How learning skills can be inspired among our trainees

Learning Skill

Learning skill is a key determinant of the LCL model. Informal education terminology, the skill of learning is a known as 'metacognition.'

Metacognition is related to:

- Person
- Task
- Learning strategy

Developing learning skill consists of three steps:

1. Identifying the Learner's Need

This step identifies the 'knowledge' or 'learning' gap

Questions to be answered:

- *What do I already know about the topic?*
- *What do I not know about the topic?*
- *What is the knowledge gap?*
- *What is the most important topic that I need to address?*

2. Developing and implementing a learning strategy
- The Learning strategy should be based on the individual learning needs
- Learning strategies are varied and unique for each learner

Questions to be answered:

- *What is the learning strategy most likely to help me to achieve the target need?*
- *What alternatives do I have? Have I selected the best strategy?*
- *What resources do I need?*
- *Have I had previous success with this strategy?*
- *What type of monitoring and evaluation is most suitable for this particular strategy?*

3. Progress Monitoring and Evaluation

The monitoring and evaluation stage allows the learner to assess whether he/she has worked to a realistic timeframe; whether the strategy and resources were effective. It is a continuous process which requires data utilization to modify and alter the learning strategy if needed.

Questions to be answered:

- What progress has been made so far?
- Is the timeframe realistic?
- Do I need to change my strategy?

What have I learned from the process that would help me in the future?

Summary:

- Metacognition is the skill of learning
- Learning Skill is an important element of the LCL Model
- Steps to promote metacognition include:
  - Helping learners identify the educational needs
  - Developing and implementing a learning plan
  - Monitoring and evaluation of learning progress

Trainer's Key Performance Indicators (KPI)	
Should be filled by trainee individually	
Trainer's Name:	
Competencies Evaluation Score: 4= Always meet expectations, 3= Usually meet expectations, 2= Occasionally meet expectation, 1= Rarely meet expectation, N/A= can't be evaluated, did not attend a session with the trainer	
Part I: Essential trainer's Skills in Classroom	**Score**
1. Opening (assess learners' needs, background, ice breaking)	
2. State objectives/ outcomes	
3. Explain the task clearly	
4. Make session interactive	
5. Providing safe environment	
6. Able to motivate the learners	
7. Applying small groups learning	
8. Controlling conflict	
9. Answering the trainees' questions	
10. Link the session to the clinical situation	
11. Good communicator	
12. Summarizing the session	
13. Feedback and reflection	
14. Time management	
Part II: Clinical Teaching	**Score**
1. Make sure that I provide appropriate communication skills with patients	
2. Assure that I use the patient-centered approach (Bio-Psych-Social approach i.e. ICE and Impact)	

3. Assure that I make appropriate case management	
4. Provide an appropriate clinical teaching	
5. Providing Mini-CEX, DOPS,CBD assessment	
6. Create a safe environment	
7. Provide a regular constructive feedback	
8. Explore my reflection	
Part III: Office Teaching (Supervision Meeting):	**Score**
1. Discuss my reflection on my learning achievements	
2. Evaluate provided evidences	
3. Helpful in guidance and support my learning progression	
4. Good motivator	
5. Create a safe environment	
6. Finding my learning gap and agree on the task	
• Developed by SBFM program in Eastern Province-MOH, Saudi Arabia, 2016	

1.4 Learners' Motivation

(adapted from Iowa State University 245/268 curriculum and instruction class (2000) taught by Barb Adams)

Motivation follows a process, which:

1. stems from stimulation
2. followed by an emotional reaction
3. leads to specific behavioral responses

Learners will be self-motivated when they:

• Know what is expected of them
• Think the effort is worthwhile

Feel they benefit through effective performance

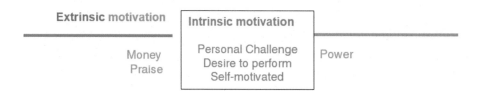

The Teacher's roles

Learners expect feedback from their teacher; the teacher needs to be aware of their verbal comments and non-verbal body language. These comments or language has either positive or negative effect on the learner's emotion and works as stimulant or inhabitant factor.

1. Demonstrate appreciation

When a learner does a good respond, the teacher should show true appreciation. Then, the good behavior or respond will be emphasized and encouraged.

E.g. of used statements:

"I appreciate that."

"I like the way you said that."

"Thank you very much for that."

2. Demonstrate empathy

Learners often give incorrect responses; in these cases the teacher should respond without discouraging the learner, ensuring that the learners feel supported, and their efforts are appreciated.

Teachers should use statements such as:

"I might make that same mistake."

"Lots of us feel that way."

"I can see how you would do that."

"I understand why you would say that"

3. Avoid unnecessary praise

A verbal motivation should not follow every positive respond. When teacher listens and gives attention, without unnecessarily giving praise. It is important that learner be able to be motivated without a stimulus of praise.

The teacher should be clear in their communications, letting learners know when they are right or wrong without stimulating any distracting emotions.

Overstatements or exaggerations should be avoided.

4. Giving praise appropriately

Learners should receive praise for good respond. The teacher should ensure that praise is distributed fairly, looking for positive in some learners where they might not be obvious.

While some learners might receive more praise for larger accomplishments than others, it is important to ensure that the lower performing learners receive regular encouragement.

The teacher should make sure that recognition is given to the class as a whole to encourage and build team unity.

The teacher should ensure not focus too much on the positive performances of one learner or group, as this can become de-motivational for others who are not performing so well.

5. Self-Assessment

It is important for the teacher to undertake self-assessment. Asking learners for their feedback "how do you describe the session" and their reflection "please tell one thing you gain from this session." In this way, demonstrate that continuous improvement is necessary.

The Learner's Role

- Learner needs to learn the importance of self-evaluation, they can do this by completing self-evaluation forms
- Keeping a journal, taking tests
- Recording revisions of work
- Asking questions, taking part in discussion

Benefits self-evaluation:

- learners are assessing what they know and what they do not know
- They are identifying what they would like to know
- They recognize their strengths and weaknesses
- They are able to set own goals

Chapter 2

Small Groups teaching and learning

2. Small Groups teaching and learning

This chapter looks at:

- The reasons for teaching in small groups
- Small group teaching techniques and method
- Tutor roles in small group teaching

Definition:

Small Groups learning is a collection of learners who interact and work together to achieve common learning goals.

- It should not be confused with lecturing to small groups.
- There is much evidence to indicate that learners learn well in small group discussion, as it leads to the "deep learning", compared to lecture-based learning which provide "superficial learning".

Small Groups are characterized by:

- Active participation
- Face to face contact
- Purposeful activity

Small group goals:

- Achieve common learning goals
- Achieve practical skills and attitude
- Support active and collaborative learning

Requirement:

- Suitable room with portable chairs
- Roundtables
- Flipchart and colored pens

Reasons for using small groups in teaching

The educational objective is the main factor, it should be one of the following to consider small groups of the teaching method:

- Achieve objectives need high order thinking skills i.e. analysis, evaluation, problem-solving
- Promote deep learning
- Teach practical skills and attitudes
- Keeping high learners' attention span
- Explore complexity and clarify doubt issues e.g. ethics issue
- Exchange individuals' experience

Tutor's Role in small group teaching:

1. Determine group's purpose and task
2. Delegate responsibilities, e.g. group leader
3. Help maturation of the small group
4. Develop group's norms
5. Resource identification
6. Crisis resolution
7. Promote learners' reflection
8. Assess group function
9. Aid group work facilitation
10. Maintain the social organization

All These roles lead to Guide learners t o Learn

Important Point (tutor role):

When a group discusses a subject, they should teach and explain the subject to other groups.

Other groups should discuss with the presented group to understand the subject and so on, to ensure the whole task is achieved by the entire groups (all learners).

Dr. Abdullah Dukhail Al-Khatami

Small Group Types

Technique is applied through systematic steps to obtain information and task.

Method a series of actions using the appropriate teaching technique to acquire knowledge and complete the task.

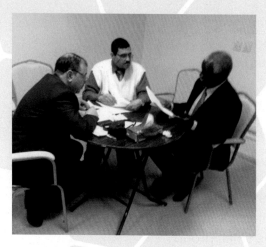

2.1.1 Brainstorming technique/method

Goal: To generate ideas

Brainstorming proceeds through two stages:

1. Ideas generation stage: this starts once the problem is stated

    - Criticism & Comments are ruled out at this stage, keeping safe-environment
    - All ideas are welcome: each idea should be written as stated by the learner without modified unless he/she agree.
    - The quantity of ideas is the aim at this stage: to collect as much as possible of ideas.
2. Ideas Combination & Improvement stage: It starts after complete all ideas.

    - Bringing together the similar ideas, then
    - Cluster ideas into groups under sub-titles, then
    - Distribute the learners into small groups, could be buzz or free discussion groups, according to the subtitle groups
    - Each group works with each to achieve the task could be in-state or scheduled a time to report their outcome to the whole group.

Brainstorming could be a technique as it goes in the below procedure:

Brainstorming Procedure

- State the problem to the whole group
- Allow a period of silent to write-down Ideas individually
- Record all ideas
- Combination and Improvement of ideas
- Discussion and evaluation then start

Brainstorming could be as a method when another technique is applied to start with e.g. buzz groups, to collect ideas during the stage one

2.1.2 Buzz Groups technique

Definition: Class Group (whole learners) divided into groups of 3-4 learners in a group to work on a task. No need for a group leader.

Goals:

- Encourage maximum participation

- Control learner's contribution
- Encourage participation of shy individuals

Buzz groups can be used for teaching a large group even up to 200 learners, but the the ideal number is 15-25.

Buzz groups technique very helpful for time-management, teacher can save time by distributing different tasks (topics) into groups. So, tasks will be accomplished in a short time. Here, each group will teach the whole group.

OR,

If a teacher has enough time, groups will discuss one task or two when completed another task could be distributed and so on.

Here, have sufficient time for discussion and have different opinions.

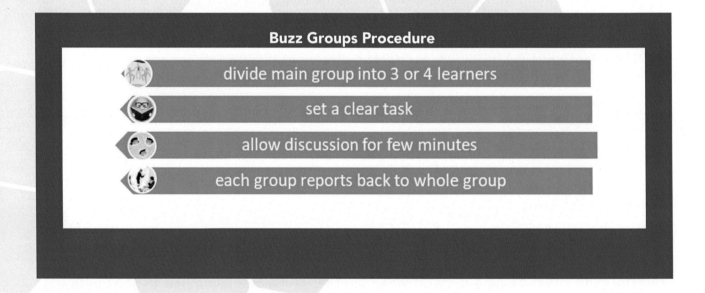

Buzz Groups Procedure

- divide main group into 3 or 4 learners
- set a clear task
- allow discussion for few minutes
- each group reports back to whole group

Snowballing technique

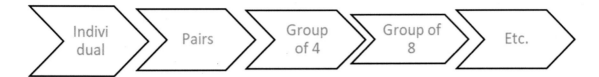

Snowballing Goals:

- Achieves agreement
- Brings all learners to approximately the same level
- Ensures participation from the whole class in discussion
- Encourages critical analysis, very important not only to sum the ideas but to discuss and criticize ideas.

Snowballing is not dependent upon the learner's preparation for its success. It depends on discussion and criticism of the ideas.

Role-play technique

Goal: Learners take on roles and act out scenarios to explore their communications skills, emotional feeling, and help modify their attitudes

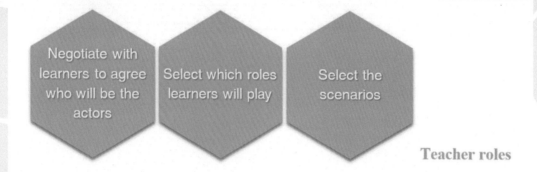

Negotiate with learners to agree who will be the actors

Select which roles learners will play

Select the scenarios

Teacher roles

Learner roles:

Important that, when finishing the scenario and the constructive feedback, the same scenario will be repeated with exchange the roles. Who was playing the role of doctor, now will play the role of the patient to learn the different experience.

Example

1. Scenario 1: Learner plays the doctor giving health education
2. Scenario 2: Same learner plays the patient role receiving health education

In scenario 1, the learner is practicing an actives/he will go on to perform in a real life situation; in scenario 2, they are exploring the feelings of the patient

Role Play Procedure

describe session nature

assign roles

ensure every individual understand their role

facilitator may play one of roles

ask Learners to mimic interaction

videotape - if possible

Constructive Feedback

Feedback in Role Play:

Crucial for affective (emotional) objectives

Important to be a constructive feedback (Pendleton style):

- Actor (doctor) be asked to describe what he/she thinks went well
  Rational: confirm and have approval for the good behavior
- Facilitator and observers highlight aspects handled well
  Rational: to highlight and emphasis on the unconscious and good behavior
- Actor describes what he/she would do differently
  Rational: to emphasis on missed points, and self-correcting for what was done wrongly.
- Group comments on what should be done in the real situation.
  Rational: to have an agreement on the future behavior (as a contract)

De-rolling

Before actors leave the session, they must de-role. Their roles may have been emotionally charged, and they need time to return to 'real life.'

By giving time for a constructive feedback and discussion before leaving place, the actor could have enough time for de-role

The facilitator is responsible for observing and helping in the de-rolling process, where other learners should not observe that.

This action will preserve the learner for contribution in the role-play learning.

Some actors are able to de-role quite easily; others require some quiet reflective time.

Free-discussion Groups technique

Definition: divided the whole learners' group into small groups, each group consist of 5 to 9 learners. One of them takes the role of a group leader to organize the work within the own group for achieving the task. Also, each group selects a presenter(s) for their task outcome.

Goal: fosters interaction and ideas exploration

Free discussion group:

- Enables openness in any topic area
- Stimulus materials may take any form
- Allows challenging for the group leader
- The teacher summarize the discussion at the end
- There is no need for clear resolution because it is for idea exploration and groups opinion of problem solution

Free Discussion Group Procedure

5-9 trainees in each group		Teacher summarizes the discussion conclusion

divide into small groups

identify discussion time

introduce stimulus material

summarise learning items

teacher facilitates discussion

by asking specific and relevant Qs

Tutorial Method

Definition:

Interaction between the teacher and small groups providing an opportunity for guidance and support.

Goal: It provides an essential strategy to support and enhance learning quality and deep learning, through probing underlying process i.e. understanding pathophysiology and mechanism of action, etc

Facilitator' tasks: Responsible for session participation, and critically probe the subject and clarify material, check progress and encourage learners to discuss material already covered.

Tutorial Procedure

Working on task: **different technique can be applied such buzz or free discussion group to discuss the topic.**

Task: **should be already explained previously in a lecture or a reading material. Prefer to present the subject in the form of a case scenario. Each scenario discusses a specific topic i.e. history, preventive measures, drug management**

Tutorials should not be turned into 'mini-lectures.' The teacher should focus on asking learners to answer questions per the task. If the learner's response is not accurate, correction should be made in such a way so as to not discourage the learner from further participation.

The teacher should take care not to focus only on issues raised by the learners but should raise further questions on the same topic to help clarify and understand the underlining process such as pathophysiology, selectivity, clinical reasoning, and comprehensive management.

Examples of case scenario:

Thyroid Disease

Scenario-1.

A 20-year-old girl comes to you. She complains of nervousness, heat intolerance and has a goiter and tachycardia.

Your colleague, who has been seeing her, feels that thyrotoxicosis is extremely unlikely in view of a history of a one-stone increase in weight over the past year."

Do you agree?
If so, what is your diagnosis?
How would you confirm the diagnosis biochemically?

Scenario-2.

A 26-year-old complains of having had a goiter for six months, a tight feeling in the neck and increasing nervousness.

O/E she has a moderate-sized goiter; hands are hot & moist; the pulse is 96.

The diagnosis is thought to be thyrotoxicosis.

She has started on Carbimazole 10 mg every 6 hours. Two months later she is no better."

Why did she not respond to carbimazole?
These examples are taken from a tutorial on thyroid disease (Paterson, 1996).

In example 1, the teacher encourages the learners to review the diagnosis to master the diagnosis criteria, achieving a high level of competency in the diagnosis of hyperthyroidism

In example 2, the teacher encourages the learners to review using carbamazepine as drug management e.g. dosage, interaction, side effects, use in pregnancy and breastfeeding, to achieve a high level of competency in hyperthyroidism management.

Seminar Method

Definition: Seminar provides an opportunity for learners to work individually and in a small group to undertake a task based on searching and report back to the whole group for a led discussion.

Seminar enhances

- **Search ability**
- **Presentation skills**
- **Critical discussion**

Teachers negotiate the learners with regards to the task to be presented. Ideally, the group will collaboratively decide on the task nature. Sufficient time (days, weeks) should be allowed between learners receiving the task and making their presentation.

Seminar presentation guidelines (Tiberius, 1990)

- Presentation work should take only 25 -50% of available time
- Feedback should be a part, if not the majority of the session
- All learners should prepare, not just the presenter

Workshop

Workshop provides an opportunity to develop skills in a simulated situation and link theory with practice (Reece & Walker, 2006)

Workshop Procedure

1. Demonstration
2. Practice
3. Assessment
4. Reapplication

2.2 Facilitator Skills

This section will focus on:

- The roles of the facilitator
- How to encourage a group
- How to maintain the group function
- Group work stages
- Facilitator skills

2.2.1 Facilitator tasks:

- Help learners to become more self-dependent
- Maintain the group function
- Ensure the group complete their task
- Ensuring success of small groups activity
- Facilitator is a major determinant of small groups success (Barrows, 1988)
- The term 'teacher' fits uncomfortably into small group work; the role of the facilitator is more effective than that of 'teacher.'

How does the facilitator encourage the group

- Encourage the group by using open-ended questions, e,g.

  Rather than saying: *"Differentiate the pain of acute myocardial infarct from the pain of an angina attack.",*

  The facilitator should say: *"Could you tell me something about the type of pain experienced during an acute myocardial infarct and the pain of an angina attack?"*

How does the facilitator maintain the group function?

Through observation, guidance, and recognize the stages of the group development:

- **Communication:** Who is/isn't actively involved? Who is talking to whom?
- **Decision making:** Who is making the decisions? How are they being made?
- **Power and influence:** What is the power pattern? Is it changing over time?
- **Conflict:** Is conflict being resolved within the group? How is it being resolved?
- **Culture:** What roles and rules have developed? What values has the group demonstrated?

2.2.2 Stages of group work (4 stages Tuckman, 1965)

The facilitator should know when he/she interfere for support, and when let group manages its situation in each stage.

In each stage let group to have time to deal and manage, if takes time ... and group couldn't move forward, then facilitator should interfere in wise and safe environment.

In forming stage: facilitator could ask "is the tasks clear? Any point need to be explored more?

Storming stage: facilitator observe who is dominant, not contribute if need a leader as in free-discussion groups should be assigned to each group by them. E.g., for the dominant, facilitator could say "good point but let us see what other want to say" without suppressing his enthusiasm.

In the case of the un-contributed learner(s): facilitator could say "let us see what is the opinion of this side" without pointing to a learner to keep safe-environment.

Be sure all reach the Norm stage.

Performing stage: facilitator should be sure what is written in the opinion of the group not only the leader or the dominant leader opinion.

2.2.3 Facilitator Roles (Skills to be mastered)

1. Establish open, trustful and supportive climate
2. Encourage safe environment

   Each learner has the right to ask and explore his/her idea without comment, criticism or arguments from others

3. Ask learners to elaborate points, e.g.

   "Could you clarify what do you mean?"

4. Explain why questions are asked

   Explain the real purpose of asking the question, i.e. is the answer unknown, is there another opinion, just checking, e.g.

   "Could you tell me what you mean, or what points led you to ask this valuable question?"

5. Probe learners' understanding of principles and concepts;

    Be sure that the learner understands the underlining pathophysiology, rationale or the purpose of the answer, e.g.

    "Could you tell me why you chose this medication to be added and how it will help?"

6. Summarize and challenge hypotheses,

    By encourage summarization and create another dimension of thinking, e.g.

    "what could be another cause?" "what is about if the patient is a pregnant?"

7. Enhance student-directed learning

    When a learner asks questions, the facilitator should encourage them to think about what the answer might be, e.g.

    "what do thing the answer is?", or search for the answer "could you look to the answer and let us know?"

8. Encourage learners to listen

    "Could we listen to Ahmed's idea" if others not listen while Ahmed is talking

9. Encourage quiet members to contribute

    Without pointing toward an individual, ask

    What does this side think the answer might be? ... looking for the quite learner(s).

10. Ensure that all learners are contributing to the discussion

    If you have a dominate learner, the facilitator could direct the question or the discussion toward other learners. If a dominant learner persists, then could say

    "thank you for your valuable contribution and let us hear from other" ... Be a smile ... to keep safe- environment!

11. Reduce tension/ conflict

    If there is an argument or a controversial point, the facilitator can intervene by clarifying the point and asking for evidence

The facilitator competencies:

- Able to assess learners ' performance and achievement
- Good in session planning
- Flexible in plan implementation
- Skilled in conducting the facilitator roles
- Empower the learners to complete their task and summaries it

Application Exercise:

Use the free discussion group technique to discuss the scenario below; the facilitator should try to apply all facilitator skills:

Case Scenario

Hamad 45 y old male presented with c/o headache on and off since 7 months back he is a known case of uncontrolled hypertension on atenolol 100 mg he gave history. of unable to relax and become worried about everything in his life he have difficulties to initiate sleep with night meres his situation worsen in last 2 weeks and he was unable to concentrate at work, and gave history of recurrent absent from work

QUESTION:

How to approach this case?

Discuss in free Group & one member should take the role of a facilitator. After discussion Group provides comments about the facilitation technique used during the Group discussion.

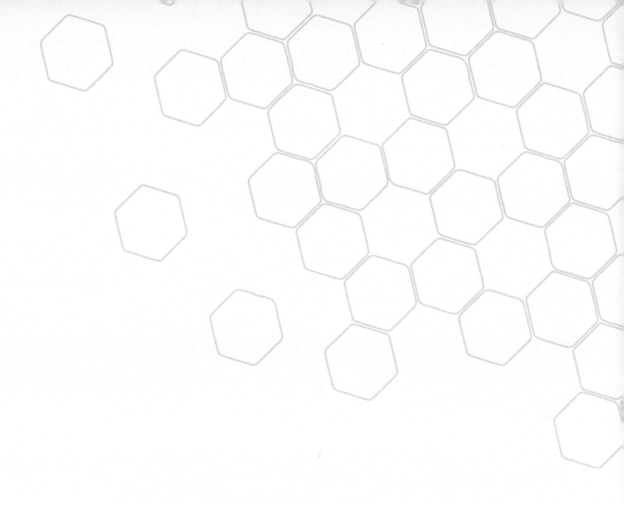

Chapter 3

Teaching Planning

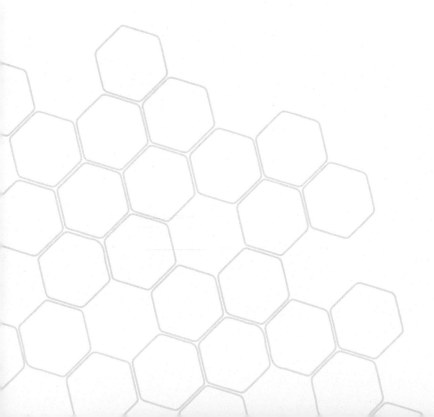

'One of the most important, as a principle of good teaching, is the need for planning. Far from compromising spontaneity, planning provides a structure and context for both teacher and students, as well as a framework for reflection and evaluation' (Spencer, 2003).

This chapter sets out the importance of teaching planning, including planning for individual sessions, looking at the requirements and benefits of planning, and the approach that should be taken.

Before teaching session, you should:

- Define your aim and objectives or learning outcomes.
- Think about the structure of the session and the timing of activities.
- Decide the best teaching and learning method to achieve the learning outcome
- List content and key topics
- Refine the lesson plan
- Identify learning resources and support material
- Ensure you have linked learning assessment for the learners' achievement.

3.1 Requirements

The essential requirements for a teaching session are:

Teaching Planning

- Planning is essential for teaching
- A flexible approach should be applied
- Teaching plan is for teaching sessions sequence

The benefits of planning are:

- Ensure effective and efficient sessions
- Enhance understanding of learners' achievements
- Excellent organisation

Planning is one of the teacher's essential Roles as a:

- Role Model
- Assessor
- Information Provider
- Planner
- Facilitator
- Resource Developer

There is no perfect approach for planning.

Flexibility is required, but the following factors should be considered in any teaching planning approach:

i.   i.   Learners' nature

ii. ii.   Resources and constraints

iii. iii.   Content- aims and objectives

I.   **Learners Nature**

Considering the previous learners' experiences is important. Understanding the content and the methods they are familiar with, will help to identify the most effective teaching content, and style could be used.

II. Resources and Constraints

Allocated time for the activity should be known: duration, which day, am or pm, who will present before and after your session.

Classroom size, content, style of chairs; suitable room with movable chairs, round tables, flip charts, and needed audiovisual.

Define the needed learning materials such colored pen, stimulant exercise, attractive scenario…

III. Content- aim and objectives

It is important to have a clear aim and measurable objectives for each session. The teaching subject will influence the choice of method used.

- **Aim** is the purpose of the activity
- **The objective** is the desired outcome for learners: each objective should illustrate and reflected in the lesson plan.
- Each session should have a part for illustration, and give a time to allow learners to apply what was taught and learned.
- In the same time has an opportunity for assessing of the learning achievement, e.g., when applying a role-play or buzz groups, it is a time for learners to apply what they learned and for learner to assess them.

GENERAL NOTE

To achieve an objective

The objective should be within the work mission which works toward the vision direction.
This objective should have strategy or strategies to be done
Each strategy should have an action plan(s) to be applied

Example

A home care unit planned to be implemented.

Vision: to be an international model for home care unit

Mission: working as a team providing an effective home care for needed patients.

Goal: to have an effective home visit care in the served area

Objectives:

      1. to establish a home visit care unit in the main centers, 4 centers, within 1 year
      2. to train a team to provide the home visit in 1 year

Strategies: (each objective need strategies to be achieved)

      1.1 identify 2 well-equipped rooms in each main center for home visit unit
      2.1 to have a well-trained team of doctor, nurse, driver in each home visit unit

Action plans: (each strategy should one or more action plan)

      1.1.1 allocate and prepare 2 rooms in a main center every 3 month for home visit unit

      2.1.1 conduct a training program every 3 month for doctor, nurse, driver for preparing them to take over the home visit care

3.2 Principles of Teaching Planning

In the planning stage consider the following items during teaching session (modified from Gagne approach, 1992):

i.   Explore learners' needs: by asking what they are thinking to gain from your session.

ii. List them in flipchart, keep it until the end of the session and review them. Is it achieved or not? Those needs which will be not covered, you can guide them from where can be got.

iii. Providing clear objectives: to be mastered in the teaching session(s)

iv. Gaining attention span: attention span usually not exceed 20minute. The teacher should concise presentation within this time, followed by small groups teaching or group to have ensured application of which learned, keep attention span, and assess the learning achievement.

v.   Presenting stimulus material: such case scenario

vi. Providing guidance: for groups' performance.

vii. Elicit performance: through illustration

viii. Provide feedback: about the learners' performance for further improvement.

ix. Assess performance: during groups work, you can assess how learners master the needed outcomes and competencies.

x.   Stimulating recall through feedback, reflection, and summarization; enforce on main points.

Also, the ASSURE model (Heinch & Molenda, 1996) as key principles for teaching planning can be considered:

1. Analysis of Learners: level, needs, their methods of learning
2. Statement of objectives- should be specific and guide teaching and learning; measurable to apply assessment tools for measuring the achievement level. Assess group work during small groups learning is one tool, even could be the only tool.
3. Selection and utilization of media and materials for teaching and learning.
4. Learners' participation: through apply small groups teaching and discussion.
5. Evaluation and revision: through summarization, feedback, reflection, and evaluate the learners' achievement.

3.3 Course and Lesson Plan

Course/Lesson Plan

Lesson plan makes teaching easy and comfortable in known and mastered sequences. One of the main outcomes of planning is to write a lesson plan format for the course (course' sessions) or a lesson. It is an important communicational tool for teachers.

Course/Lesson Plan Content

1. Topic title: This will presumably the subject suggested by a course outline, a textbook, or a state curriculum guide.
3. Goal and objectives: a list of your learning intentions in broad and specific terms

3. Content outline of the material to be covered in as much detail as you feel is needed; this should help clarify the subject and aid you with the sequencing and organization.

3. Learning activities: this should cover teacher and students activities and should include introductory, developmental, and culminating activities. When arranged into a series of daily lessons, these will lead to the desired learning outcomes.

3. Resources and materials: a list of materials to be selected and prepared for the session(s).

3. Evaluation: use a technique that determines how well students have mastered the intended learning outcomes of the lesson. The facilitator can assess the learners during the small group learning through observation, contribution, feedback, reflection. These should be planned and prepared for instruction.

Lesson Plan Format

A lesson plan should provide the necessary structure to a lesson but should be general enough to allow for flexibility. Suggested basic lesson plan format:

1. Course/ Lesson Title
3. Introduction (set induction): an activity used at the beginning of the course/ lesson to attract learners' attention and interest.

3. Objectives: the specific learning intent for the day, selected from the unit plan. These objectives should determine the sessions' activities.

3. Session format contains:

- Session's number, title, Speaker (facilitator), date, duration
- Table has these column titles: Subject duration, name, teaching method, resources needed

  - Closure, the lesson wrap-up activity: summary, feedback, and reflection

Example: Course Plan format

Title: Biopsychosocial approach and Doctor-Patient relationship

Aim: Improve PHC physicians' ability to explore patients' perceptive and apply the biopsychosocial approach effectively.

Objectives:

1. To improve doctor-patient consultation skills to achieve case-control status.
2. Define the patient' perception, stress & chronic cases.
3. To learn "ICE & Impact Technique" to provide comprehensive care.
4. To define the relationship between doctor and patient, factors affect Doctor-Pt relationship.

Session 1: Bio-Psychological Consultation Model

Duration: 2.5 hours

Activity time	Subject	Teaching Method	Resources
10 mins	Learners' Needs	Q & A	Flipchart
20 mins	Bio-Psychological Consultation Model (Traditional+ ICE and Impact technique)	Interactive Lecture	PowerPoint
15 mins	Break		Coffee Room
30 mins	Illness behavior: Patients' perspective	Interactive Lecture	PowerPoint
50 mins	Bio-Psychological Approach	Buzz Groups (Role Play and observer)	Suitable Room/ Flipchart
10 mins	Summarise		
15 mins	Feedback and Reflection		
30 mins	Break		

Session 2: Doctor-Patient Relationship

Duration: 2 hours

Activity time	Subject	Teaching Method	Resources
10 mins	Background assessment	Q & A	Flipchart
30 mins	Doctor-Patient Relationship: types and affected factors	Interactive Lecture	PowerPoint
60 mins	Patient Interview	Role Play	Suitable Room
10 mins	Summarize and conclusion		
10 mins	Feedback and Reflection		
CLOSE			

EXERCISE:

In buzz groups, design a lesson format for a session of 1.5 hours, and your plan should include:

- Title
- Aim and Objectives
- Instructor' name(s)
- Time
- Topics
- Teaching method
- Resources

3.4 First day of Class

It is the stressful day for both learners and teacher. It is natural for both to feel anxious, and uncertainty on the first day of class.

To manage these, it is important to implement the following principles:

1. Handle administrative matters
3. Put learners at ease: at the beginning of a teaching course, better to start in a semi-circle class to make discussion open without a barrier. Each learner Introduce his/herself. Then, explore the learners' needs.

3. Create a relaxed and safe classroom environment: each learner has the right to ask and clarify any point, no criticism, each one has an own opinion can be expressed with objection from other learners. The teacher has the right to guide the discussion toward the objectives of the course in encouraging way.

Let Learners know what you expect from them, and what they can expect from you: by express the objectives, tasks, and requirements.

Chapter 4

Presentation Skills

Dr. Nada Al-Bunaian

Definition: The presentation is a type of communication in which you transfer your ideas to a group of people in various speaking situations such as lecture or meeting settings.

Components of Presentations

- **Presenter**- the person who communicates with the audience and delivers a message.
- **Audience**- the group of individuals who receive the presenter's message. The audience participation will depend on their background knowledge and experience
- **Message**- It could be a verbally, non-verbally, with/out using an audio-visual aid
- **Method**- the way of delivering the message by the presenter which is either directly or remotely e.g. Online, webinars
- **Implémentation**- how the presenter presents the message

The main stages of the presentation:

1. Preparation for presentation: the stage before presentation time in which you work on your speech (see lesson plan)
3. Presentation skills: the art of providing your ideas to a group of people.

Presentation skills are mandatory in every field not just in medical education. Presenters could be reluctant because they concern about criticism or confrontation. These fears can be addressed through proper preparation.

4.1 Preparation for presentation

It is a crucial and important step. Good preparation will increase confidence and support good time management during the presentation. Items needed to be considered in the development stage:

1. Objectives
2. Subject
3. Knowing your Audience
4. Be familiar with Place and setting
5. Time of Day
6. The presentation's duration
7. Develop and organize the presentation material

Your presentation should give a clear and well-structured message, you should know what you want to say, and in what order.

Organizing your presentation material

Brainstorm- generate ideas

- Note down all the ideas you would like to talk about; don't worry about placing them in order at this stage
- Choose the main points
- Identify your beginning, middle and end- Introduction, Main Content, Conclusion
- Introduction should inform the audience of your subject matter, setting out the main points
- Main content will deliver the detail around your main points, giving them substance
- The conclusion will summarize your messaging

> Always remember that time and timing is important; ensure you have allocated the correct amount of time to each point
>
> Your main points should be arranged logically and should be supported through discussion and engagement with the audience

Presenting your ideas

- Identify how you will present the main content, using text, diagrams, images, visual aids
- Think about how you might simplify the text through the use of diagrams for examples

Finalize your introduction and conclusion

- To attract your audience, the introduction should give them a preview of what you will be talking about
- Explain the importance of this subject matter
- Keep it simple; make it stimulating
- The conclusion should summarize the main content, and lead to a solution, or next steps

Editing your content

- Use appropriate language and familiar words
- Use accessible and easily understood words and avoid technical or obscure words
- Keep your sentences short with simple structure, so your audience focus on what you are saying rather than reading from the slides
- Use metaphors to help your audience to understand and retain your ideas, e.g., figures, charts, tables, etc
- Identify tools to keep your audience's attention e.g. use videos, case scenario, games, etc.
- Ensure there are no spelling mistakes in your presentation

4.2 Presentation Method

- **Full text**- use the whole text in front of you during the presentation. It is an important "do not let this distract you from your audience." Avoid reading directly from the text, and instead, use the text as a trigger for your message.
- **Cue-card**- write key points and triggers, or cues, for the next points; the key points can include supportive notes. It helps you talk about each point NOT just reading the pre-determined text. A set of numbered cards can be an effective way of organizing your thoughts and time-management for the presentation.
- **Mind Maps**- using diagrams contain the main points, ideas and tasks, showing connections between each
- **Visual Aids**- this is the most commonly used method of delivering a presentation. It should be used if it is necessary to keep the audience attention and support the most important points' delivery. You should not use visual aids to demonstrate technical skills that, will distract the audience. It helps to provide a clear and a concise message.

Most commonly used visual aids are:

- Whiteboard
- Flip chart
- Presentation software, e.g. PowerPoint
- Handout

4.2.1 Using whiteboard

Whiteboards are helpful in developing an explanation, listing headlines, drawing flowcharts, and recording audience comments and ideas during brainstorming sessions.

Handwriting should be clear, aligned horizontally, and large enough to be read by all. Use non-permanent markers.

If you are going to use an interactive whiteboard, you should make sure that you are familiar with the technology before using it "live" with your audience.

4.2.2 Using flipcharts

A flip chart provides an excellent tool for presentations. It is easy to use, accessible and cheap. It is perfect for brainstorming, spontaneous explanation, and summarization.

When using flip charts, you should:

- Arrive early to position the flip charts and make sure that there are enough charts and working markers
- Stand next to flip charts facing your audience while presenting

- Use only blue and black markers to be clear for those who sit at the back, using red markers only to highlight already written points
- Make your letters clear and large- about 2-3 inches tall
- Keep your handwriting aligned horizontally; you can draw horizontal lines in pencil

4.2.3 Using video

The video provides the best media for training purposes, in particular, teaching communication skills and the demonstration of examination and procedures.

Ensure computer is connected to the projector, speakers and, the internet if needed

Video may be played directly from YouTube, DVD, or can embed into a PowerPoint presentation.

4.2.4 Using Powerpoint

PowerPoint is most commonly used. It could prove a most efficient way of delivering a presentation.

You should ensure that your PowerPoint does not distract your audience their ability to engage with you as the presenter.

You should pay careful attention to:

- The structure of your presentation
- Font and font size
- Colors and background of the slides
- Use of figures, tables, diagrams, and graphs- these should be easily understood
- Clarity, simplicity, and conciseness of your slides-
- Avoid multiple colors, backgrounds, animations, and clip art

Right Slide structure

Demonstrate one point at a time:

- Helps the audience to concentrate on what you are saying
- Prevents them from reading ahead
- Helps you keep your presentation focused

Caution when designing slides

- Animations can be fun and engaging, but you should take care not to overuse them
- Use animation consistently throughout your presentation
- Avoid multiple directions for text entry on animated slides
- Avoid attempting too much impact with animations, e.g. avoid text movements that are very slow
- Do not use distracting animation, swivel or bouncing
- If you have a laser pointer, use it sparingly, e.g. for emphasizing a point, avoiding pointing which can be distracting

Slide fonts

Use standard fonts (San Serif type styles, e.g. Arial, Calibri); avoid italic or connected letters as this strains the audience's eyes

Avoid capitalization, except for emphasizing a point

Be consistent with the font type

- Use 44-50 point font for the main title, and 32 point font for slide title
- The minimum point you should use is 24 point font (preferably 28)

Slide colour

- Make sure that the font color is contrasted with the background color
- Be consistent in the use of color throughout your slides
- Use different color or bold font to emphasize a point
- Avoid red and green colors, as people who are color blind, will have difficulty reading them
- Make sure that the color contrast is not distracting and is relaxing to the vision

Slide background

- Keep your slide background simple and attractive
- Be consistent throughout your slides
- Avoid dark background in a well-lit room
- Use light background and dark font color, particularly if you are not sure about the room lighting
- Avoid using backgrounds with different colors

Figure, table, graph, and photo

- Use figures, tables or graphs to clarify and substantiate information for easy visualization of data
- Make sure that this fits with message
- Always title figures, tables, and graphs with a clear font
- Mention the copyrights for ethical consideration

Graphs provide a better visual than flow charts or text:

- Easy to present data
- Easy to visualize

You should always ensure your graphs are titled.

The following example will show the difference between displaying data in a table and a graph:

It is clear that the data in the table is difficult to trace, is crowded and takes the time to understand the information, and therefore, the message. The graph, however, sets out the data in an easily accessible format.

The photo should relate to the subject, not repeated the text content.

It could be a break between 2 sub-titles

It should not be too much

Instructions for attaching a video to your presentation

1. Make a link to a file that opens in an external player
2. Attach (embed) a video onto the slide:
   a. Write a word or insert a figure to link it to the video
   b. Highlight the word or the figure and right-click on it and chose hyperlink, a gray window will appear

   c. Insert the browser link to the video's web page (if you are linking to a video on-line) or enter the file address (if you have the video on your computer)

   d. When you double click on the word or figure it, the video will start immediately

Including activity slides

Sometimes it is helpful to use slides to notify the audience of the time/event, e.g. a coffee break

Conclusion slides

The last slide in your presentation should include the following:

- Summary of the main points
- Question and answer
- Take audience feedback and reflection
- Close the session by thanking the audience

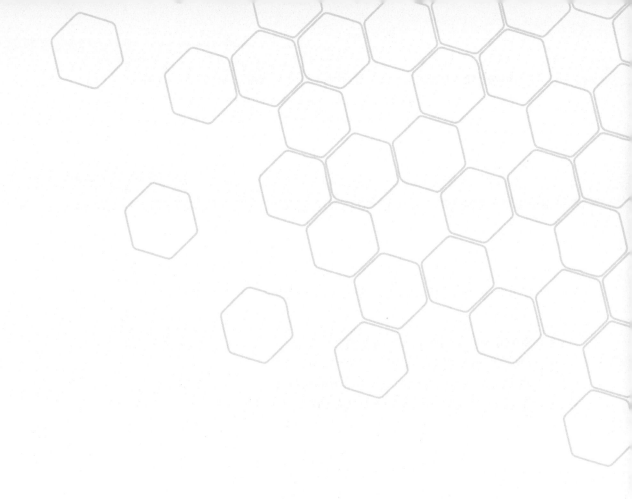

Chapter 5

Clinical Teaching Skills

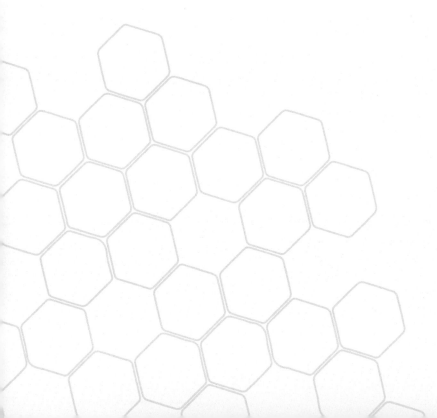

Clinical teaching is at the core of teaching and learning in Medicine, involving patients and their problems and illness. It is a demanded task.

Definition of clinical teaching:

In modern teaching, the clinical teaching is a form of social interaction between preceptor (clinical teacher) and trainees with defined goals around the patients' problem, NOT only around the disease, as in the traditional teaching.

It is an opportunity to share information, demonstrate a technique, clinical observation, feedback, and reflection through case discussion.

Effective clinical teaching improving with regular practice when combined with feedback and reflection

Clinical teaching goals:

1. Enhance the trainee's knowledge and skills
2. Improve practice efficiency and effectiveness
3. Promote clinical independence
4. Prepare trainees for optimal patients health care
5. Become a competent and collaborative clinician
6. Able to be an efficient in time management

5.1 Clinical Training Delivery

This section looks at the precepting model for clinical teaching delivery. What's required to identify and understand the learning needs? It applies an effective and efficient clinical teaching approaches, which prioritizes the trainees' need. It provides an effective use of clinical teaching time that achieves the most impactful and successful outcomes.

Clinical teaching models

Three emerging models for the clinical teaching, the preceptors should be aware and master them to be an effective and efficient in their duties, as outlined by Morton-Cooper and Palmer (2000). They formulated into 3-steps for clinical teaching by Stalmeijer et al. (2010) based on the principles of cognitive apprenticeship (Collins et al., 1989). These models determined by the level of the trainee.

Step 1: Modeling model:

Preceptor works as a skilled **role-model.** Trainees learn by observing their preceptor's practice. It is appropriate for the beginner trainees to be familiar with their proposed tasks.

   - Aim: facilitate trainees learning, and modeling.
   - Clinical teacher' responsibilities:

   1. Create a safe learning environment is a basic for feel free to ask questions and seek guidance.
   2. Expected to be a good role model
   3. Demonstrate relevant skills

Step 2: Coaching Model

Preceptor carries out as an **instructor and coach** who shows and assists the trainees in achieving a set of competencies. Its process is a collaboration between trainee and preceptor. There is a space for the trainees to practice certain competencies under supervision. They have a chance to receive feedback on their performance and express their reflection about what they did and what they have learned.

This model also called *"competence-based model"* and fits for the junior trainees till they master the required clinical competencies. In medical branches there 6-comptencies needed to be learned (see 5.2).

Step 3: Reflective practitioner model

Preceptor plays the role of the critic friend or mentor. It is a based on articulation and exploration of the trainees' clinical reasoning in a constructive feedback. It is appropriate for the senior trainees who already pass the stages of modeling and coaching. Its process is based on stimulation of self-directed learning through collaboration and partnership in the learning process between preceptor and trainees.

Its aim is to guide and support learning through define the learning gaps, identify an appropriate learning process, and to assess the learning achievement. In this model, the case-discussion could be conducted at the end-clinic. It is the main model used in the supervision meeting, office discussion, and portfolio assessment.

5.2 Teaching Clinical competencies

	Step1: Modeling Step2: Coaching	Step3: Directed learning
Clinical competencies	**Junior Trainee**	**Senior Trainee**
1. Appropriate Communication Skills	• Basic communication skills: welcoming, rapport, verbal, non-verbal, open questions, empathy, summary, follow-up.	add: •dealing with difficult cases •breaking the bad news
2. Patient-Centred Approach	• bio-psychosocial approach **bio:** traditional history, physical exam **psycho-social:** explore patient' perception through ICE and impact technique (patient's idea and concern about the presenting symptom(s), the expectation of the visit, impact of presented symptom(s) on sleep, performance, and relationship. •state the problems list	add: • appropriate investigation • discover stress resources and hidden agenda • shared care • continuous care • collaborative care
3. Professionalism	• well-commitment and punctuality • respect colleagues and staff • doctor-patient relationship skills • reflective skills • time management • inter-professional relationship skills	add: • familiar with system and process • advocates patients' need
4. Selectivity	• prioritize the problems • appropriate differential diagnosis	• add: • selective and efficient in data gathering • focused and targeted questions to reach the real diagnosis, management

Clinical competencies	Step1: Modeling Step2: Coaching Junior Trainee	Step3: Directed learning Senior Trainee
5. Clinical Reasoning	• promotes critical thinking • interpreted data • approach: probabilistic reasoning	add: • able to make decisions with limited information •Problem-solving skills • Approaches: probabilistic, casual, deterministic reasoning

Clinical Medicial Competencies:

Clinical competencies required are well-defined by the Royal collage of family medicine of Canada. These competencies are the Patient-centered approach, Communication skills, and Communication skills, selectivity, clinical reasoning, professionalism and procedure skills.

1. **Appropriate Communication Skills**

The doctor/trainee should apply the appropriate communications skills as the situation requires- building rapport, exploring the patient's agenda, verbal and non-verbal communication, eye contact, empathy.

2. **Patient-centered approach:**

It is achieved by applying the **bio-psychosocial approach** when interviewing the patient.

Bio-: covered through the traditional approach (sign and symptoms, physical examination, investigation, and management).

Psycho-Social: covered through applying the Idea, concern, expectation, and impact on sleep, performance, and relationship (ICE-impact) technique. If one of these six questions are affected, then it is important to screen for psychological disease such as depression, anxiety, etc.

The aim of applying ICE is for exploring the *hidden agenda* "Ask About the presenting symptom."

I idea *"what do you think the cause of your presenting symptom?"*

C concern *"why do you worry from this presented symptom?"*
E expectation *"what do you expect from me to do for your presenting symptom?"*

The aim of asking about the impact on patient's sleep, performance, and the relationship is exploring the stress presence, at least for the last two weeks, and its severity.

Sleep;

- *"when you put your head on the pillow, Do you get to sleep easily?"* "Early insomnia" happen in the mild-moderate case.
- *"when you get to sleep, is it interrupted?"* happen in moderate-severe case
- *"Get up early morning with a difficult to sleep again?"* means late insomnia, happen mostly in severe case
- *"do you have a prolong sleep?"* usually happen in atypical depression

Patient's performance: compare your performance with before symptoms. When there mark decline, moderate to severe case.

Patient's relationship; how is your relation to surrounding people. Usual effected person complain from they changed not like before. Mostly happen with a severe case.

3. **Professionalism:**

Professionalism is behavior based upon the master of a complex of knowledge and skills, which used in service of others. Acting professional is a necessary complementary skill for competent practice.

Professionalism has **four elements**: Doctor-patient relationship skills, inter-professional relationship skills, time management, and reflective skills.

4. **Clinical reasoning skills:**

This dimension deals with problem-solving skills, making series of inference about health stat, which applied through 3 clinical reasoning approaches:

I. **Probabilistic Reasoning**

Depends on determining 'event probability, e.g., the likelihood of disease, chances of successful treatment & prognosis after treatment. It based on known disease prevalence and other statistical data about the disease. Exemplified by usage of qualifying terms

– *"What is the most likely diagnosis?"* Prognosis….

II. **Casual Reasoning**

Its process establishes relationships between more than two observed events.

Examine: whether the occurrence of an event (A), can be explained by event (B). It depends on an understanding of the pathophysiology and therapeutic knowledge to explain the patient's clinical events.

III. **Deterministic Reasoning**

It is based on ambiguity about action. Its encountered in the form of the clinical algorithms and flow charts. It is a technique of applying **'if and then.'**

Teacher emphasizes possible ambiguous situations when such approach not practical or feasible, e.g., if this asthmatic patient presents with high fever and rhonchi in the chest auscultation, *"what is the possible diagnosis."*

EXERCISE "in buzz groups."

Discuss which clinical reasoning approach could be used to reach the case explanation or diagnosis, and then determine the appropriate management?

Case 1.

A 25-year-old lady presented in ER with tongue protrusions, muscle rigidity, torticollis for short-term history. No history of chronic diseases, last two have had attack gastroenteritis which was managed as an ambulatory case. How do you explain the patient's case?

Case 2.

50-year-old diabetic patient during an interview for his follow up felt drowsiness and then the loss of consciousness. What is the most likely cause?

Case 3.

If a newborn baby presents with symptomatic hypoglycemia, the treatment should be …? Explain the rationale for administration of IV glucose

5. Selectivity:

This dimension skill concerns about setting priorities, knowing when to say something and when not to. It facilitates to gather the most useful information without losing time on less contributory data, doing something extra when it will likely to be helpful, distinguish emergent from elective, select and modify treatment to fit patient need or situation.

Example

A 35-year-old gentleman presented for a health check-up. No complaint, blood transfusion, or contact with jaundice pt.

-What is the selective question would you ask the patient to reach the most likely diagnosis?

	Result	Units	flags	Range
Glu	88	Mg/dl	-	70-110
Chol	252	Mg/dl	HIGH	5-200
Tri	161	Mg/dl	-	50-200
HDL	41.09	Mg/dl	-	35.00-65.00
ALKP	90	U/L	-	40-120
ALT	86	U/L	HIGH	0-50
AST	35	U/L	-	5-40
GGT	111	U/L	HIGH	12-64
BUN	17.2	Mg/dl	-	7.0-20.0
Creat	1.1	Mg/dl	-	0.5-1.4

ANSWER:

You should be asking the patient whether he drinks alcohol. The cue for this would be the high GTT.

5.3 Practical teaching according to Resident level

Dr. Shatha Alzuhair

Trainees' Level

I.   Modeling and Coaching Stages (junior trainees):

1. Trainee most often assigned one to one sessions with a preceptor in a clinic.
2. The trainee is responsible for assessing the vital signs and review the patient file before the interview.
3. Trainee starts by establishing a good rapport, welcoming the patient, and introducing his/herself.
4. Patient interview 'bio-psychosocial approach' according to the "Disease-illness model" observed by the preceptor; this should take around 10-15 minutes

Preceptor writes comments during a patient interview without interruption unless patient Safety is affected.

5. Trainee proceeds to examine the patient once permission is taken
6. Discuss the case with the preceptor, before the management stage,

   • What is the most likely diagnosis?
   • Evidence of conclusion?
   • Why is a decision taken?
   • Investigation required and why?

7. Management part is the responsibility of the preceptor.
8. The preceptor should provide constructive feedback (see feedback part):

II. Self-directed learning (senior trainees):

1. The trainee is often charged to a clinic.
2. Responsible for assessing the vital signs and review the patient file.
3. Establish a good rapport by welcoming the patient and introducing him/herself.
4. Patient interview 'bio-psychosocial approach' according to the "Disease-illness model."
5. Focused examination once permission is obtained; this action takes about 10-15 minutes.
6. Trainee documents the problems list
7. Formulate the management plan.

The trainee should spend around 5-10 minutes discussing the case with the assigned preceptor to identify the learning gaps. Preceptor better to use the "five micro-skills steps for clinical teaching" method.

If the clinic moves smoothly, two options for the time of the cases discussion, according to the clinic crowdedness:

- One-on-one over cases, where case discussion conducted after each case, role modeling and coaching, or
- Case rounds discussion: "on-end clinic discussion": where around group discussion includes trainee(s) and his/their preceptor meet to have feedback and reflection. Trainees also will have a chance for exchanging their experiences. This technique is preferably for those trainees who are competent enough to run the clinic as safe doctors. It takes about 30-45 minutes.

- **Challenge your trainees...... but show them how to succeed Trainees need to believe the goals are achievable**

- **Make learning FUN! ... Engage the trainees!**

Why is case discussion important for trainees?

- Trainees need to hear feedback about their performance
- They need to know how they are doing at one level before progressing to the next.
- To define their learning gap(s), strengths, and opportunities for improvement.

5.4 General Teaching Principles

Key to successful clinical teaching are the following principles:

I. Active participation
II. Focusing attention
II. Scope broadening of patient specific information
II. Meeting individual needs
II. Regular feedback & assessment

Identifying the trainee needs

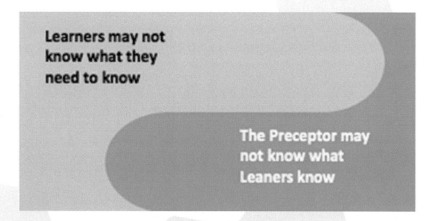

Four possible scenarios express the trainee's need in the clinical teaching shown below (Whitman & Schwank, 1984):

I. Shared Knowledge

• Preceptor knows the trainee's knowledge
• Preceptor's role is to enhance this knowledge by:

  • Reiteration (repetition)
  • Validation
  • Identification of key learning issues

II. Hidden Knowledge

• Preceptor doesn't know what knowledge the trainee has
• Preceptor's role is to explore the trainee's knowledge by asking about their:

  • Experience
  • Interest
  • Strengths

• Preceptor then prioritizes objectives and direction

III. Known Need

• Preceptor knows that the trainee lacks in knowledge and skills
• Works both on these defects to build them

IV. Unknown Need

• Both preceptor and trainee don't know the trainee's knowledge and learning needs
• Provide a task, observe and assess to define the trainee's level.

Precepting

Precepting is an educational interaction between trainees and a preceptor in a clinical setting. It depends on the preceptor's interest to guide and train through the gradual promotion of trainees.

Precepting aim to develop self-confidence trainees who can deploy their newly acquired skills and behaviors independently.

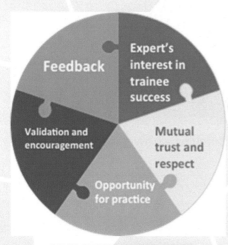

FIVE-STARS PRECEPTOR

1- Preceptor's interest to graduate self-dependent trainees

2- The relationship between trainees and preceptor based on a mutual, trust, and respect

3- Preceptors should create opportunities for their trainees to practice what they learned

4- Trainees should receive regular validation and encouragement for their learning

5- Preceptors should provide regular a constructive feedback for their trainees' performance

5. Preceptor role:

• Explore trainee's knowledge and experience
• Identify known and unknown needs by enhancing reflection

• Promote and allow space for application of knowledge within the context of patients' individual physical and psychological needs through a constructive feedback.

6. Clinical Teaching Guidelines

• Learn about useful teaching models

- Recognize "how clinical reasoning process can be taught effectively during clinical teaching."

- Identiefy common mistakes during clinical teaching

- Use case-based teaching scripts to provide:
  - Short clinical vignettes of similar cases
  - Efficient use of limited teaching time
  - Understanding of trainees' action in advance enable teachers to respond quickly

7. Clinical Teaching Process

Clinical Teaching Implementation through two simultaneous processes: image

These two processes are achieved simultaneously by:

I.   Targeted questioning
II. Review trainee records
III. Educational intervention, demonstration, feedback
IV. Increasing shared knowledge and minimizing unknown knowledge

Preceptor's challenge is to support trainees to learn the most important and most relevant topics in a short period.

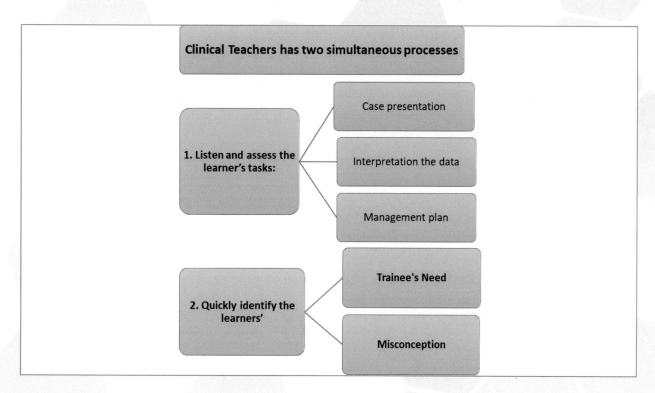

5.5 Constructive Feedback in Clinical Teaching

Feedback should be specific statements about the directly observed behaviors. It uses non-judgmental language and balance descriptions of the learner's strengths and areas for improvement. It is identifying the learning gaps.

It takes about 10-15 minute.

1. Teacher observes:

   - Learners' presentation
   - Clinical examination
   - Clinical reasoning process (the core point)
   - Management decisions
   - Providing feedback to learners

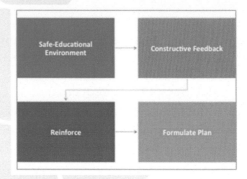

2. The purpose of feedback in clinical teaching:

   1. Improve confidence and clinical performance
   2. Improve the quality of performance
   3. Important to avoid trainees' misconceptions
   4. Natural agreement between trainee and preceptor is essential for effective feedback

Feedback should be:

- Constructive and Not-personal
- Well timed and given in privacy
- Based on trainee's level
- Consistent with trainee's needs and goals
- Focused on the trainee's performance
- Collaborative with open questions
- Given using relaxed body language
- Given in a safe environment

Feedback Problems:

- Fear of giving criticism
- Insufficient time allocated for discussion and completing assessment form

---

Feedback Contents

- Constructive feedback:

---

1. Start with learner's self-assessment what went well
2. Reinforce what the preceptor think went well
3. Learner self-assessment about what could be improve

- Preceptor reinforce the right actions

–important points for providing specific feedback
–NOT for all points
–to review understanding & feeling to these points
–How to be done in appropriate way

- Formulate

- Specific & realistic plan with clear directed goals

Learning video:

https://www.youtube.com/watch?v=PRIlnUAKwDY

Constructive Feedback Steps:

- Trainee interviews patient and completes the assigned task. - 50% of time (10-15min)

- Preceptor allows the trainee to starts with his/her self-assessment, through asking two questions:

  - "What went well?" its purpose is to enforce the good things
  - "What could be improved?" to allow the trainee to correct mistakes or remember forgotten issues.

- Then, Preceptor reinforces positive points and specific areas for improvement, through two comments - 20% of time

  - • "Points went-well?" receptor reviews understanding and feeling and reinforce good achievement. By asking "what do you think is things you do well?"
  - • Then, preceptor reinforced the well-done.
  - • "Areas for improvement" select 2-4 critical areas for improvement, not more even if present. Ensure that, the trainee well understand them with empathy demonstration, for remembering and mastering these points.

3. Formulate specific and realistic plan with a clear, directed goal to improve further performance with mastering the discussed areas - 10%

Constructive feedback should be used to formulate a precise and realistic plan with clear and focused goal

---

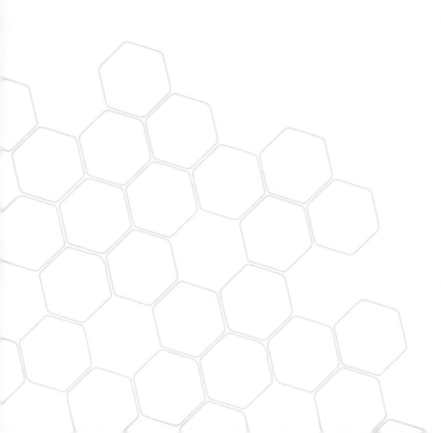

Chapter 6

Five-Micro Skills for Clinical Teaching

Five Micro-Skills for clinical teaching (One Minute Preceptor)

It is described by Neher et al. as "A Five-step "Microskills" Model of clinical teaching. Journal of the American Board of Family Practice. 1992 (5):419-424.

Most clinical teaching takes place in the context of a busy clinical practice.

Micro-skills enable preceptor to be an efficient assessor, instructor, and feedback provider.

This model is used primarily when the preceptor knows the case needs.

Five Micro-Skills for clinical teaching

It is one of the several models and has shown to be a better studies model:

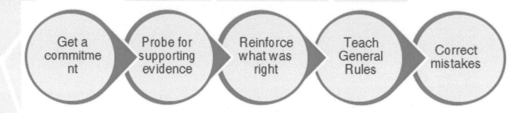

Teaching Reasoning during Case Presentations

This process mirrors the preceptors' minds. They first focus on diagnosing the patient's problem, then on diagnosing the learner's needs, and finally on providing targeted instructions.

The micro-skills facilitate this instructional process. The first two micro-skills, Get a Commitment, Probe for Supporting Evidence, diagnose learner knowledge and clinical reasoning.

Reinforce what was right, teach General Rules, and Correct Mistakes offer tailored instruction.

MicroSkill 1: Get a Commitment

Trainee's task is to articulate his/her diagnosis or plan; the following questions are helpful in this step:

I.   What are the likely possibilities in this patient?
II. What is the most valued information obtained?
II. What would additional information be helpful to know?

The preceptor should resist commenting and allow the trainees to express their diagnosis/plan.

Trainee expects some guidance from the preceptor.

The rationale behind keep resistance to commit is to allow the trainee to determine their learning requirements and define their gaps.

Without this, learning can be misdirected and time may be spent discussing issues which do not support the actual learning needs.

MicroSkill 2: Probe for Supporting Evidence

Trainees express and clarify why they say that commit (diagnosis, investigation, management …). Therefore, they articulate their diagnosis or plan; the following questions are helpful in this step:

1. Why did you consider this as the most diagnostic possibility?
2. What were the main findings that led you to your conclusion?
3. How does this information help you to narrow down the diagnostic possibilities?

Also in this step, the preceptor should resist making comments to evaluate trainee's knowledge and clinical reasoning capabilities, and identify his/her knowledge gap.

1. *Cue*

   In the case of discussion, trainee usually looks to preceptor either confirm or suggest an alternative. The preceptor may or may not agree should resist commenting trainees know more or less than they do, and risk

2. *Preceptor*

   Before offering your opinion, ask trainee for his/her evidence.

   Consequence

   Then, ask what another choice could be considered with supporting evidence.

3. *Rationale*

   Trainees proceed with problem-solving logically from their knowledge and database.

   Preceptor asks about trainee's thought processes, allows both to find out what known and to identify the learning gap.

   Without this information, the preceptor may assume targeting instruction inefficiently

MicroSkill 3: Reinforce what was Right

By reinforcing what was right, should provide positive feedback about trainee's performance.

It is important for trainees, they may underestimate their reasoning process or not recognize their positive performance. Therefore, make it a conscious and improve the chances of permanent retention of information.

The reasoning process is significant, and without highlighting it, the trainee may perceive good response as "pure luck" and not recall this experience in the future.

Providing positive feedback before correcting mistakes will maintain trainee's ego and self-respect, making the mistake-correction (the next step) more acceptable.

AVOID COMMENTS SUCH AS:

"You are right. That was a wise decision." "You did that preparation very well."

Micro-Skill 4: Teach General Rules

What are "General Rules"?

When we talk about "general rules," we refer to all and any rules which can be useful in future cases. Each patient is unique, although opportunities and advice arise for other situations usually happen, phrase it as " when this happens, do this … ".

General rules enable the trainee to connect episode specific learning experiences to other cases with the help of some general principles.

General rules should be targeting the learner's level.

Instruction is both more memorable and more transferable if it is offered as a general rule.

EXAMPLES:

"If the patient has depression as result of using b-blocker or oral contraceptive pill. You have to stop these medications before taking a decision of antidepressant start."

Micro Skill 5: Correct mistakes

Providing constructive feedback with recommendations for future improvement is a critical element of the Teaching and the Learning processes-

Remember, trainees expect to make mistakes, if not corrected there will impact on future practice and patient care. The mistake has a risk to be repeated.

Allowing trainees to correct themselves is an important part of this process. It makes the scenario more acceptable and supports them in identifying their needs and learning gaps.

The preceptor should focus on providing the transferable General Rules, and then provide feedback to the trainees about their performance.

EXAMPLE:

"I agree that the patient is asking for sick leave, but we still need to take a history and examine them before assumption."

APPLICATION EXERCISE:

Case scenario: A trainee presents a young lady with a cough

1. Get a commitment

Preceptor: "What do you think is going on?"
Student: "I think this patient has bronchial asthma."

2. Probe for supporting evidence

Preceptor (nodding): "What clinical findings led you to that conclusion?"
Student: "She has symptoms of short breath, cough, and wheezy chest."

3. Reinforce what was right

Preceptor: "That's an excellent summary. It shows you've taken a good history, performed focused physical examination. I agree with your diagnosis."

1. Get a commitment

Preceptor: "Now- how do you want to manage her asthma?"
Student: "I want to start on bronchodilator and steroid inhalers."

3. Reinforce what was right

Preceptor: "I agree that we should start an inhaler. Remember, we need to know in which severity level she is before taking a decision"

4. Teach general rules

Preceptor: "The general rule to learn from this case is that we need to know in which asthma severity level before starting medication."

5. Correct mistakes; identify learning gap

Preceptor: "Please look up how we could define the asthma severity level? So, we may discuss it at the end of the clinic.

Learning videos

http://www.youtube.com/watch?v=9N904yuf7a0&feature=player_detailpage

Chapter 7

Work-based Assessment

Dr. Abdullah D. Al-Khathami , Dr. Abdulaillah ALQurashi

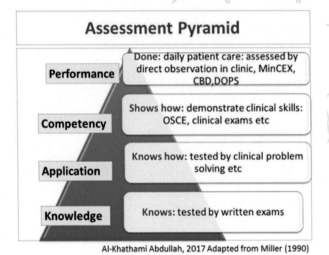

Assessment Pyramid

Performance	Done: daily patient care: assessed by direct observation in clinic, MinCEX, CBD,DOPS
Competency	Shows how: demonstrate clinical skills: OSCE, clinical exams etc
Application	Knows how: tested by clinical problem solving etc
Knowledge	Knows: tested by written exams

Al-Khathami Abdullah, 2017 Adapted from Miller (1990)

This section looks at Work Based Assessment (WBA) tools, focusing on the following areas:

1. The teaching approach
2. Feedback as part of Work Based Assessments
3. Mini CEX, DOPS, and CBD Assessment Forms

Goals of Work Based Assessments:

- Assess the trainee's progress over time, observing their performance in areas of professional practice
- Form part of the ongoing instructional process
- Support and enhance learning improvement over time (Shepard, 2000)
- Include self-evaluation, and the setting of action plans
- Identify trainees' need at an early stage
- Provide regular feedback, agreeing how professional needs will be met
- Encourage the practice of reflection to support trainee learning and development

Formative Assessment

Formative Assessment allows preceptors to be trained on the purpose and process of the observation and feedback strategy. (this is why WBA forms were initiated).

Key Performance Indicators (KPI) for the Trainee's Clinical Competences	Date:
Trainee's name:	Trainer's name:
Please score the trainee from 1 to 5 for each items(1)- is least (5) is max - N/O no observed (keep empty if N/O)	

Appropriate Communication skills: Trainee able to	Score
1. Welcoming and establish rapport (patient & family)	
2. Communicate at patient education level	
3. Showing empathy and caring for the patient	
4. Utilize appropriate verbal and nonverbal skills	
Total Communication Skills	

Patient centered approach: trainee able to	
1. Define real reason for patient attendance	
2. Explore ICE and impact (sleep, performance and relationship)	
3. Screening about mental illness (depression and anxiety)	
4. Evaluate the back ground context (past medical ,surgical, family history… etc	
5. Assess red flags and risk factors	
6. Demonstrate physical examination and detect the finding	
7. Clarify the natural of the disease to the patient	
8. Provide disease prevention and health promotion	
Total Patient centered assessment	

Professionalism : trainee able to	
1. Doctor-patient relationship and	
2. Interpersonal good relationship	
3. Trainee's self-development (reflective skills)	
4. time management	
Professionalism Score =	

Selectivity : trainee able to	
1. Able to be selective in asking the patient	
2. Prioritize problem list	
3. Demonstrate prober use of diagnostic tests	
4. Appropriate use of pharmacological therapy	
5. Appropriate use of referral	
Selectivity Score =	

Clinical reasoning : trainee able to	
1. Able to utilize clinical reasoning hypothesis(probabilistic, casual, and deterministic) **Score=**	

Procedure skill: trainee able to	
1. Perform specific procedure (diagnostic and management) **Score=**	
KPIs score	

Trainers' comments:	
Areas of strength:	
Areas for improvement:	

• **Developed by SBFM program in Eastern Province-MOH, 2016**

Key Performance Indicators (KPI) of Training Centers	Training Period:			
Please score the trainee from 1 to 5 for each items(1)- is least (5) is max - N/O no observed (keep empty if N/O)				
Evaluation items Centers	Training center-1	Training center-2	Training center-3	Training center-4
1. Trainer punctuality				
2. Trainer discussion				
3. Trainer gives feedback and comment				
4. Trainer applies assessment methods				
5. The training-period is helpful				
6. Nurse is available as needed				
7. Cases varieties and availability				
8. Availability of resources				
9. Safe-learning environment				
Total score				
• Developed by SBFM program in Eastern Province-MOH, Saudi Arabia,2016				

Formative Assessment Methods

1. Mini Clinical Evaluation Exercise (Mini CEX)
2. Case Based Discussion (CBD)
3. Direct Observation of Procedural Skills (DOPS)
4. Clinical Work Sampling (CWS)
5. Blinded Patient Encounters (BPE)
6. Clinical Encounter Cards (CEC)
7. Multi-Source Feedback (MSF)

The more commonly used methods are MiniCEX, CBD, and DOPS.

The provision of the structured feedback based on observed performance is the core to the purpose of this type of assessment. Trainees are expected to be evaluated several times across a range of situations, and with a range of patients- by different faculty members; this enriches the learning and evaluation process.

The general rating scale used is shown here:

- Trainee do the selected task ~15 min
- Assessor scores the trainee's performance
- Preceptor provides a constructive Feedback 5-10 min
- Allow trainee to provide own reflection
- Working together for identifing the learning gap

7.1 Mini-CEX

Developed in the US (Norcini et al., 1995), the goals of Mini-CEX are:

- Provides a teaching opportunity which enables the assessor to share their professional knowledge and experience.
- Allows for multiple direct observations of real patient situations, assessing:
  - Communication skills
  - History taking
  - Physical examination skills
  - Professional practice
- Guides trainees' learning through the provision of structured feedback.

A key benefit of MiniCEX is that it provides strong internal consistency and is replicable (Kogan et al., 2003), with high validity to discriminate senior from junior residents.

Inter-rate reliability and scoring among levels of assessors can vary.

Approximately four encounters are considered a reliable and sufficient to achieve an accurate outcome. Mini CEX is correlated with written in-training examinations and the results of the Royal College oral examination.

- trainee engages in the work-based encounter
- perform the clinical task: focused history, physical exam, diagnosis,and/or management
- preceptor observes and scores the trainee's performance
- preceptor provides a constructive feedback
- in a collaburative agreement with the trainee identify learning gap and improvement plan

Each technique is scored using a 9 point rating scale:

Unsatisfactory (score 1-3)

- Trainee is unable to perform a procedure
- Trainee has poor technical ability
- The result gives cause for concern
- Trainee needs to repeat the procedure

Satisfactory (score 4-6)

- Trainee meets the standard overall and is technically competent

Superior (score 7-9)

- performance is above expectation
- assured competent and sufficiently technically
- proficient to teach the procedure

Active videos examples

  WPBA – MiniCEX at

http://dai.ly/x5sapio

password is TOT.Book

7.2 Direct Observation of Procedural Skills (DOPS)

DOPS allows an educational supervisor to observe a trainee undertaking a practical procedure directly, and to make judgments about specific components of the observed procedure and grade the trainee's performance in carrying out the procedure (Wilkinson et al., 2003).

DOPS was originally developed at the Royal College of Physicians in London (Wragg et al., 2003). There is evidence to show the validity and reliability of observational assessment tools.

DOPS is considered to be reliable only when at least three supervisors have assessed at least two procedures each.

Developed in the UK, DOPS scores trainees' performance using a 6 point rating scale:

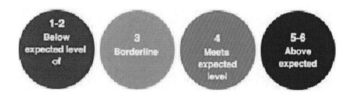

7.3 Case Based Discussion (CBD)

CBD was established by the American Board of Emergency Medicine, 1983.

CBD Purpose- why we need CBD

- Systematically assesses the trainee's performance and explores professional judgment in clinical areas, especially trainee thinking (Clinical Reasoning) and problem-solving ability
- Guides the trainee's learning through structured feedback
- Provides valid, reliable and provide excellent feedback, which is effective and efficient in changing practice.
- Should be triangulated with other methods of assessment
- Utilizes professional judgment, which is the ability to make holistic, balanced and justifiable decision in situations of complexity and uncertainty

CBD is highly correlated with:

- Standardized patient exam
- Chart audit
- Written exam
- Oral exam

Medical Record Keeping

- Should be legible, signed, dated and appropriate to the problem
- Understandable about and in sequence with the entries
- Helps the clinician using it to give effective and proper care

History Taking

- Trainee discusses how they understood the patient's story through the use of further questions
- Conducted examination as suitable for the clinical problem
- Clinical assessment was performed from which further action was derived

Clinical Findings and Interpretation

- Trainee discuss the rationale for the required investigations and necessary referrals
- Shows understanding of why diagnostic studies were undertaken, including the risks, benefits, and the relationship to the differential diagnosis

Management Plan

- The trainee should discuss the rationale for his/her management plan including the risks and benefits.

Professional Qualities

- Trainee should discuss patient care as recorded, demonstrating respect, compassion, empathy, established trust, and confidentiality
- Consider the ethical approach and awareness of any relevant legislative frameworks
- Trainees has insights into their limitations

Overall Clinical Judgement

- Trainee should discuss own judgment, synthesis, caring and effectiveness for the patient case at the time that the record was made
- Able to define, with the support of the assessor, areas of strength, improvement and planning needs
- He/she can provide self-reflection for further personal development.

Ask-Tell-Ask Feedback Method

<u>Ask</u>

- To verbalize trainees' thoughts on what they did well, what needs improving
- Validate things trainee has identified that are accurate and expand your perspective
- To come up with strategies for improving performance by focusing on alternatives rather than on one solution
- Give student time to think and respond

<u>Tell</u>

- Explain what you observed, "I observed …"
- Balanced feedback both positive and corrective elements
- React to the learner's observation

<u>Ask</u>

- Ask about trainee understanding and strategies for improvement with questions such as: What do you think?" Do you agree? How do you feel about …?
- Commit to monitoring improvement together

Conclusion

WBA form is applied to:

- Observer trainee performance
- Provide a constructive feedback
- Allow trainees to learn from their performance and correct their self by self- Reflection
- Help to define individual learning Gap
- Assign related & particular task to be fulfilled

Key Performance Indicators (KPI) of training centers Training Period:					
Please score the trainee from 1 to 5 for each items(1)- is least (5) is max - N/O no observed (keep empty if N/O)					
	Evaluation items Centers	Training center-1	Training center-2	Training center-3	Training center-4
1.	Trainer punctuality				
2.	Trainer discussion				
3.	Trainer gives feedback and comment				
4.	Trainer applies assessment methods				
5.	The training-period is helpful				
6.	Nurse is available as needed				
7.	Cases varieties and availability				
8.	Availability of resources				
9.	Safe-learning environment				
Total score					
· **Developed by SBFM program in Eastern Province-MOH, Saudi Arabia,2016**					

Chapter 8

Companion of Office Supervision
meeting & Portfolio assessment

This chapter provides:

- A clarification of portfolio types with emphasis on the section-type portfolio;
- Explain the theoretical basis of educational supervision in different learning contexts: office, clinic, and classroom.
- Scope of the educational supervision; process of educational supervision; assessment of supervision

Portfolio:

The term portfolio is derived from a Latin word porter (to carry) and folium (leaf, sheet). It is defined as *"A collection of a student's work, which provides evidence of the achievement of knowledge, skills, appropriate attitudes and professional growth through a process of self-reflection over a period of time"* (Davis et al., 2009).

Portfolio Types:

If portfolio is only a collection of what were done, it would be Log-book. Portfolio is more than this – it contains what were done plus reflection.

There are different portfolio types:

1. **Learning Portfolio:**

   It includes personal reflective responses to learning experiences. It has three fundamental components: documentation, reflection, and collaboration. These combined reflective documentations may be discussed for the purpose of assessment and feedback. It provides a critical opportunity for purposeful, mentored reflections and analysis of evidence for both improvement and assessment of learners' learning achievement (Davis et al., 2001a, O'Sullivan et al., 2004).

2. **Assessment portfolio:**

   It includes the collection of the most typical work -which reflects the learner's best work on certain themes over a period. Observations test scores, anecdotal notes, evaluations, etc. (Pitts, 2007). It judged when the trainee achieves needed competencies.

3. **Selection Portfolio:**

   It is a task-based or training period task-based portfolio. The trainee provides his/her reflections about the different training events during each training period e.g. during introduction training period, hospital rotation period.

The purpose of such method is to assess the achievement of intended learning processes; hence, trainee collects multiple drafts that represent a chronology of progress in his/her learning achievement through assessing his/her reflections. These reflection's forms have the content of the selection Portfolio.

It allows the supervisor to assess the trainee's critical thinking, clinical reasoning, and problem-solving skills, interpreting and analyzing information. The best forum, where all these attributes are discussed with a supervisor in an office supervision meeting.

Framework (scope) of Supervision meeting:

Trainees should present their reflections related to the activities they had during a period after the last meeting.

Supervisor uses a template for each a training period to organize and conduct the supervision meeting; to assess the trainee's reflections structuralrly.

For each activity's reflection, the supervisor should assess and support the trainee's achievement in 3 domains: identify the learning gap(s); help to choose an appropriate learning process to fulfill this gap; then assess the achievement in the next meeting.

It facilitates the communication between supervisors and reminder for next meetings, and as a tool to visualize the covered learned areas.

In general, trainees have classroom and clinical sessions. In the classroom session, they have to reflect on the educational activities that they had attended and kept these reflections as a content of their portfolio. For the clinical sessions, trainees provide their reflection about their performance on a selected case(s) (selected by the trainee). They should collect a minimum number of case-based discussion (CBDs), Directly Observed Procedural Skills (DOPS), and Mini Clinical examination (Mini-CEX), as needed in the curriculum.

They should reflect on these events and receive feedback from the assigned trainers. These documentations should be kept as a part of the portfolio contents.

Discussion of the clinical documentations could be given to the registrar without discussed in the supervision meeting because they were discussed before. OR, could be discussed in the supervision meeting, depending on the time, the ability of the trainers, the benefits may be raised. However, if it's re-discussed, it should be taken from a different angle, to define a learning gap, monitor the trainee as a family physician.

DIFFERENCE BETWEEN DISCUSSION AFTER PERFORMANCE IN-CLINIC AND OFFICE:

In Clinic trainer discuss the performance issue

Where in office trainer discusses the clinical reasoning behind the decision-making.

Example

Supervisor Meeting
[Portfolio Assessment]

Supervisor's Name: **Date:**

Trainee's Name:

Meeting: ☐ 1   ☐ 2   ☐ 3

	FM-2 Rotation		
	HDR	CBD	Logbook
Assessment Tools	F2*	F3	F5
Required Cases (RCs)	1/2wks	1/2wks	#cases
	Overall Assessment		
Achieved RCs (yes, Partial, or No)			
Score#			

N/B Discussion should cover 1-2 reflections, chosen by the trainee, to define 2-3 Learning Gaps in each meeting. Not necessarily identify all gaps in one meeting.

#Rank the candidate from <u>1-5</u> based on completion of the following Assessment Domains:

- present the meeting ….. Score (1)
-Identify learning needs ….. Score (2)
- Search for evidence ….. Score (3)
-Achieve the identified needs ….. Score (4)
-Did extra effort as a specialized physician ….. Score (5).

N.B: Kindly submit this form to the program Registrar after completion

Trainee's Signature: **Supervisor's signature:**

Designed in SBFM in Eastern Province-MOH Saudi Arabia, 2012

Example

Tasks Form
[Supervision Meeting Follow-up Report]

Supervisor's Name: **Date:**

Trainee's Name:

Keep this report in your portfolio document for next follow-up meeting

What do you want to learn more?	How will you learn?	Assessment	Evaluator
Meeting1: • • •		☐ Complete ☐ Partial ☐ Not done	
Meeting2: • • •		☐ Complete ☐ Partial ☐ Not done ☐ Incomplete	
Meeting3: • • •		☐ Complete ☐ Partial ☐ Not done ☐ Incomplete	

designed in SBFM in Eastern Province-MOH Saudi Arabia, 2012

Supervision meeting Process:

Each trainee is assigned to a supervisor to meet regularly in an office every 2-4 weeks and lasts for 30-45 minutes.

Supervisor uses the non-clinical time to review trainees' portfolio and assess trainee's reflections on the program activities. This dialogue encourages trainees to be involved in promoting their reflective practice in a safe environment.

It's imperative to make trainee feel safe because the conflicting dialogues can affect their learning achievement.

Supervisor assesses trainees' reflections on critical incidents by skillfully asking questions; consequently, trainees revise their learning events on which they have reflected.

The trainee then defends their work by answering through logical reasoning and showing different pieces of evidence in the form of articles, guidelines, videos, etc.

After their oral defense, the supervisor and trainee are in a position to judge trainee's performance based on the assessment template as mentioned above. Usually, supervisors also involve trainees in decision making.

That promotes reflective practice and self-directed learning attributes among trainees. While defending, if further gaps are identified, then these will be documented on "Supervision Meeting Follow-up" report which will be re-assessed in the next supervision meeting.

Trainee Support:

To ensure a high quality of learning and achievement during all components of the training period. Each trainee should be assigned to a Supervisor and Mentor (faculty advisor).

Supervisor

- Supervisor assesses the trainee's progression through review his/her learning achievement over a training period (portfolio assessment).
- Supervisor facilitates the learning process by evaluating the trainee's portfolio for identifying learning gaps and guide for an appropriate learning method.
- So, Supervisor Meeting Roles: help the trainee to identify the learning gap, aid to choosing an appropriate learning process to fulfill this gap, then assess the achievement in the next meeting.
- Learning gap(s) should not exceed three gaps in any given point of time, to be accessible achievement.

- Assigned supervisor should follow the trainee for at least three months, then changing is preferably for further experience exchange.

Mentor

- The mentoring partnership is described as a contract between two people sharing experiences and expertise to help personal and professional growth.
- A mentor is the one who has vast experience, talent or professional standing and promotes the career of a mentee.
- Mentoring is beyond supervisory mentoring not necessarily taking place in the work environment.
- Assigned Mentor should follow the trainee for at least one year for building real trust.
- Key to Success:

    - Respect
    - Clarify expectations and needs
    - clear goals and an action plan
    - Manage the mentoring process by making sure of meetings

Mentor Rules and Responsibilities:

- Meet with the mentee at least once per 2 or 3 months
- Mentor Roles, assume four main coaching roles:

    - Teacher: Assisting the mentee's goals and plans to achieve them.
    - Counselor: Discussing work-related concerns impeding performance or career growth.
    - Guide: Sharing personal experience.
    - Challenger: Providing objective and honest feedback.

Mentee Rules and Responsibilities:

- Take the initiative and proactive in his/ her career development
- Keep the mentor informed of mentoring progress through mail/phone/in-person etc.
- Conduct open and honest discussions with the mentor
- Keen to have a feedback
- Develop an Individual Developmental Plan
- Meet with the mentor regularly at scheduled meetings

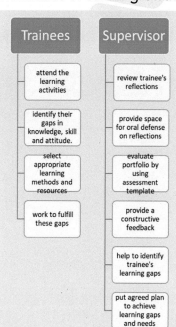

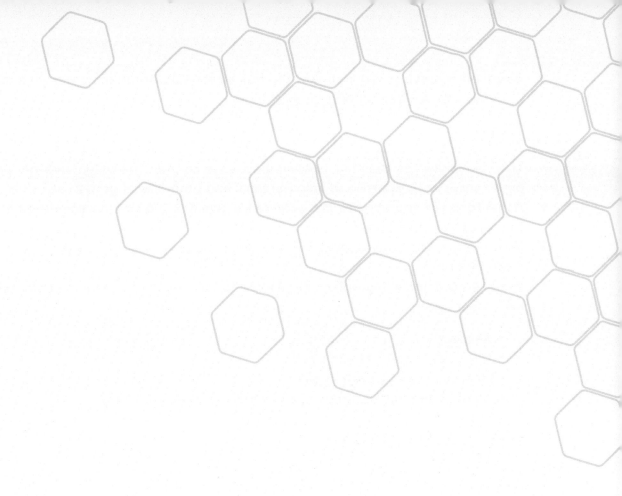

Chapter 9

CanMEDS Roles in Medical Practice

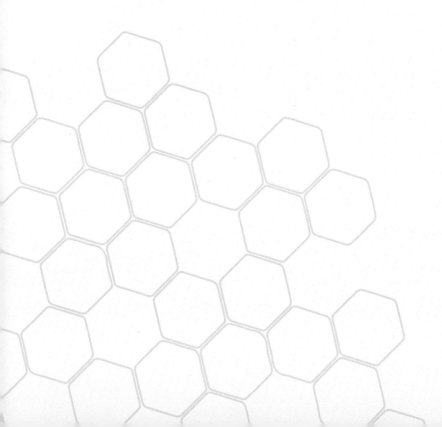

Training of the Trainers: Clinical Teaching Skills

CanMED Role Purpose

- Define necessary competencies for all areas of medical practice
- Provide comprehensive foundation for medical practice.

How to apply CanMED Roles in training programs?

First, we should know when we talk about Role, we talk about action (verb) not objective of a person. For more explanation: when a trainee did an action reflects the expert role, not mean he/she become expert. But, the action e.g. collect needed data was expert role, despite when the trainee interpret the data incorrectly, the trainee didn't reflect the role of expert here and so on…

Our aim is providing the trainers with needed skills to be able to teach and assess their trainees in the view of CanMED Roles.

Outcomes:

1. The candidates will be recognize and apply the CanMED Roles in their daily practice as trainers.
2. They will be master how can adopt and assess MED Roles among their trainees

Medical Expert Role:

- It is an important of integrating all the six roles of CanMED
- It required for the Selectivity and Clinical Reasoning competencies
- It is reflected in the following actions:
- Providing a high quality, safe, and patient centred care

  o have effective clinical skills and professional values
  o Be able to collect data and correctly interpret them
  o Understand his/her expertise limitation
  o Built the decision based on:

1. Best practice and research evidence
2. Consider their patient circumstances and patient's preferences
3. Consider the resource availability

Scholar Role:

- It is a lifelong learner component

- safe learning environment

- Search for Evidence-based practice

- Critical appraisal

- Research findings

Scholar Role Requirements

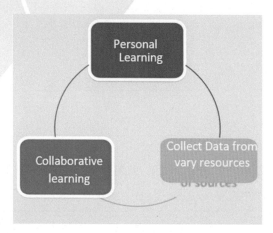

Communicator Role

- It is required for the communication skills and patient centred approach competencies
- Focus on the interaction between the physician and patient,
- also interaction with patient's family in purpose of collect data

Collaborator Role

- Address handovers and care transferred to another physician or health care professional
- Collaboration amongst physicians
- When involve the patient's perspective or their families in shared decision-making
- Extend collaboration beyond context of the heath care team
- Communication with other colleagues forms a part of the Collaborator Role

Leader Role

- Emphasis on leadership skills to improve health care
- Promote patient safety
- Develop skills to achieve balance between the professional practice and the personal life

Health Advocate Role

- Contribute to improve health care through understanding the needs.
- Speaking on behalf of others for their values
- Supporting resource mobilisation for effective change and help others
- Improving quality of clinical practice and organisations for serve internal/external costumers

Professional Role

- it reflects when person master the art or science
- In crude clinical competence providing an optimal care
- Commitment to ongoing professional development
- Adhere to the ethical standards, honesty, respect
- Respect the conflicts of interest

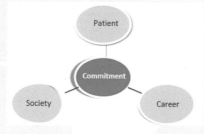

CanMED Role	Action Description
Medical Expert Role	• Provide high-quality, safe, pt-centred care • Able to collect, interpret data • Decision-making based on EBM • Consider pt's circumstances, preferences, resources availability • Understand expertise limitation
Scholar Role	• Lifelong learner component • Utilize Safe learning environment • Searching for EBM • Applying critical appraisal • Looking for research findings
Communicator Role	• interaction between Physicians & patients and their families • Emphasize on communication & Pt-central approach competencies
Collaborator Role	• Address handovers & care transitions • Collaborate among physicians • Pt shared in decision-making • Extend beyond H care team
Leader Role	• Emphasis on leadership skills to improve health care • Promote patient safety • Develop skills to balance between professional practice & personal life
Health Advocate Role	• Contribute to improve H. care through understand needs • Speak on behalf of others when needed • Resources mobilization • Improve quality of practice& organization
Professional	• Commitment and punctuality • Mastering practice for offering H care • clinical competences providing optimal care • Adhere to ethics, honesty, respect • Respect conflicts of interest

CanMED Roles Scenario

Khadija is a 65 years old diabetic patient came to her family physician's clinic, Dr. Faisal. Her blood sugar is not controlled. Oral medication reached the maximum dose. She well-follow her doctor advices and instructions.

Upon these information, Faisal decided to change her medication to insulin injection. Therefore, he review the updated guideline and his decision was supported to start injection. Dr. Faisal took a very detail history for her social situation from the patient and her relative. The management plan was discussed with patient, and she couldn't able to use insulin injection and nobody could give her it in regular base but, her relative agreed to bring her to the center for injection.

Faisal discuss the issue with PHC director and reached to give her in insulin daily in the center with well-organized procedure. The director suggested for Dr. Faisal to form a team to serve such patients. Faisal started to select a nurse and wrote a plan and procedure for the new service.

Could you kindly illustrate the CanMED roles through the above scenario?

Use the below table:

CanMED Role	Example
Medical Expert	
Scholar	
Communicator	
Collaborator	
Leader	
Health Advocate	
Professional	

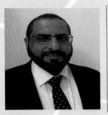

CERTIFICATE VITE

DR. ABDULLAH DUKHAIL AL-KHATHAMI

MBBS, ABFM, FFCM(KFU), MSc Medical Education (Cardiff University-UK)
TQM, Diploma/MSc PMHC (Nova University Lisbon- Portugal)

TITLES

- **Consultant, Family and Community Medicine**
- **Specialist in Medical Education, PMHC, TQM**
- **Affiliated Consultant trainer in Maastricht University**
- **International Expert Consultant- Primary Mental Health Care– Wonca**

Address
KFHU-P.O.Box 40248
Al-Khobar -31952
+966-505845821
mabna@yahoo.com

I- PRESENT POSITIONS

2016- Now	Director, Primary Mental Health Initiative Program-MOH
2003 – Now	Supervisor, the Primary Mental Health Program in Eastern Province-MOH.
2010- Now	Trainer for TOT Courses at the National level – SCFHS
2012- Now	CBAHI - Primary Care Surveyor – Saudi Arabia
2016-NOW	Vice-Chair Wonca- Working Party Group on Mental Health -EMRO

Previous Roles/positions

II- PRESENT POSITIONS

May 2014- 2016	Chairman of the Trainer Unit in Family Medicine-Saudi Commission of Health Specialties-Saudi Arabia
Feb 2014-2015	Chairman of Training Committee - Saudi Diploma Joint Program in North Border Area.
2002 –2004	Director, Community Mental Health Services (CMHS), Al-Amal Complex for Mental Health, Dammam, Saudi Arabia.

2003 – 2006	Trainer, Saudi Commotions of Medical Specialists joint program in King Faisal University, Dammam, Saudi Arabia.
2006 – 2007	Coordinator Between Health Provider Sectors, Joint Family Medicine Program, Eastern Province-MOH, K S A.

III- INTERNATIONAL PROFESSIONAL ROLE / MEMBERSHIP

	enrolled Date
WHO Guideline Developing Group Member - for management of physical health conditions in people with severe mental disorders.	9-10 May 2018
Vice-Chair – Wonca Working Party Group on Mental Health	2013-2016
Vice-Chair – Wonca Working Party Group on Mental Health-EMRO	Nov 2016-Now
Affiliated Consultant trainer in Maastricht University	April 2016-Now
International Expert Consultant- Primary Mental Health Care– Wonca	Nov 2014-Now
Chairman, Trainer Unit Family Medicine – SCFHS	Jun 2014
WHO mh GAP Action Plan 2013-2020 A presenter of Wonca in the annual WHO Mental Health GAP Forums	October 2013, 2015, 2017
Coordinator- Between Wonca Working Party Groups AND Research Group	Jun 2013
Vice-Chair – Wonca Working Party Group on Mental Health	2013-2016
Member – WONCA - Education interest Group	2013
Member – WONCA - Research Interest Group	2013
Member - Mediterranean Regional Mental health Advisory Group (EMERO)	2012 –Now
Member – Local Saudi Family Medicine Board Committee, Saudi Commission for Health Specialties (SCHS)- Eastern Province.	2012 –Now
Member – Local Family Medicine Diploma Committee- (SCHS), Eastern Province.	2010 - Now
Member – Scientific National Committee of Primary Mental Health-M.O.H	2008 – 2010
Member - Postgraduate Family Medicine local committee, Saudi Council for Medical Specialists, King Faisal University - Eastern Province	2005 – 2006
Member – Local Community Mental Health Committee in Eastern Province (M.O.H)	2004-Now
Member - World Organization of Family Doctors (Wonca) Working Party on Mental Health	2004- Now
Editor - Journal of Mental Health in Family Medicine/WONCA, WHO	2004- Now

IV- PROFESSIONAL AFFILIATIONS

Member - Saudi Society of Family & Community Medicine.   2002

Member- American Academy of Family Physicians.   2003

Member- Arab Healthy Water Association (AHWA).   2005

Member - Saudi Psychiatric Association   2006

Member – EMRO Psychiatric Association   2015

V- REFERENCE FOR MEDICAL & SCIENTIFIC JOURNALS

King Abdulaziz City for Science & Technology - Review Committee, Riyadh, Saudi Arabia.

Saudi medical Journal - Review Committee, Al-Khobar, Saudi Arabia.

Journal of Family & Community Medicine - Review Committee, Al-Khobar, Saudi Arabia.

International Reference Group for WONCA- Primary Mental Health Care in PHC - Review Committee.

Academic Supervise for postgraduate Family Medicine dissertation - Saudi Board certification- Dept. Family and Community Medicine KFU. Subject "Prevalence of Mental Health problems among PHC patients in Dammam city-SA"

VI- AS THE TRAINER FOR TOT COURSES

HAD CONDUCTED SINCE 2008 IN TOTAL 36 TRAINING COURSES

1- Effective Teaching Skills & Portfolio Assessment Course (3days): Total 238 trainers were trained conducted 12 courses.

2- Clinical teaching skills & Work-based Assessment Course (2days): total112 trainers in Aseer region, Arar, Internal Defense Hosp Dammam, Madina Munora, and Makkah

3- Comprehensive TOT Course (5days): Total 250 trainers were trained in Makkah region, 23 in Riyadh (Shamaisi Hospital), KFH in Riyadh, SPFM-Riyadh-MOH (in 2 periods), Arar (in 2 periods), Gryate, Jouf.

4- CanMED Roles in Practice and assessment (1day): 185 trainers and resident, Eastern Province-MOH, Asser, Makka, KSU-Riyadh (in 2 periods), PGFM Riyadh (in 2 periods)

   Conducted 6 courses

VII- INTERNATIONAL CONFERENCES & SYMPOSIA – SPEAKER

No.	Title, Place & Date	Duration
1.	Trail of Primary Mental Health Care in Eastern Province, Saudi Arabia, Tripoli, Lebanon, September 2004	3 Days
2.	Implementation & Evaluation of Mental Health Training Program for PHC Physicians, 1st International PHC Conference, Abu Duabi, UAA. Jan. 2006	3 Days

3.	Community Mental Health – Saudi Arabian Pilot, Florence, Italy, Aug 2006	5 Days
4.	The Implementation & The Out-come of Primary and Community Mental Health Program, Saudi Innovation Conference, Newcastle-UK, May 2007	2 days
5.	Appling Communication Skills in Patients' Interview in PHC , a Training Course for Family Physicians, Cairo, Egypt, November 2008. a trainer	2 days
6.	Family Health Profile/ Prescribing/ Referral System in Family Practice, Cairo, Egypt, May 2009. a trainer	2 days
7.	International Transcultural Psychiatry Conference , Ranchi, India: 24-25 Sept 2011	2 days
8.	Does intervention training Course improve the PHC physicians' satisfaction and welling to work in PHC centers?. Wonca-2013, Prague, Cz 25-29 Jun, 2013	5 days
9.	Wonca Working Part group on Research meeting and workshops, 24 and 26 Jun 2013, Prague CZ.	2days
10.	Wonca Working Part group on Mental Health meeting, 25 Jun 2013, Prague CZ	1day
11.	International Forum on Innovation in Mental Health , 3-4 October 2013, Lisbon, Portugal	2days
12.	WHO Mental Health Gap Forum: Special Focus on Mental Health-Action Plan 2013-2020, 7th October 2014, Geneva	1day
13.	Learning to work in Integrated Care training professionals for a new service model: Saudi-Portugal Collaboration, 28-30 April 2015, Lila France	3days
14.	Depression and Anxiety among Hypertensive and Diabetic Primary Health Care Patients: Could sleep disturbance be used as a screening tool for Depression and Anxiety?. Wonca-EMRO Conference, Abu-Dubai, 2-4 March 2017	3days

VIII- RESEARCH AND PUBLICATION:

Several researches and contributions were done as illustrated below.

A. Scientific Books

4. **Integrating mental health into primary care:** A global perspective World Health Organization and World Organization of Family Doctors (Wonca) 2008,   Printed in Singapore. (Contributor)
5. **Companion to Primary Care Mental Health**; 2012,Radcliffe. (Co-Author)

A. Scientific Articles:

6. The Effect of Diabetes Mellitus on the Presentation of Depression in a Primary Care Population in Saudi Arabia, Master Dissertation to Obtain the Master degree in Primary Mental Health, Nova Medical University, February 2018

7. Mona Ahmed AlShaikh, Abdullah AlKhathami. Evaluation of Physicians' Communication Skills at Primary Health Care Centers, KSA. INTERNATIONAL JOURNAL OF SCIENTIFIC RESEARCH. 2017; VOLUME-6 (4): 611-618.

8. Abdullah D. AlKhathami, Mohamed A. Alamin, Areej M. Alqahtani, Wafaa Y. Alsaeed, Mohammed A. AlKhathami, Abdulazeez H. Al-Dhafeeri. Depression and Anxiety among Hypertensive and Diabetic Primary Health Care Patients: *Could sleep disturbance be used as a screening tool for Depression and Anxiety.* Saudi Medical Journal, 2017; Vol. 38 (6): 621-628

9. Rawaf S, Qidwai W, Khoja T, Nanji K, Kurashi N, Alnasir F, Al Shafaee M, Al Shetti M, Bashir M, Saad N, Alkaisi S, Halasa W, Al-Duwaisan H, Al-Ali A, Farahat T, Tarawneh M, Al-Khathami A, Abutiheen A, Iqbal Azam S, Swaka A. New Leadership Model for Family Physicians in the Eastern Mediterranean Region: A Pilot Study Across Selected Countries, 2017. J Fam Med - Volume 4 (2): 1107 page 1-8. www.austinpublishinggroup.com

10. Al-Khathami, A. Leadership in Postgraduate Family Medicine Training Programs: A "Steps-Model" Implementation in Eastern Province-MOH Saudi Arabia. Middle East Journal Of Family Medicine, 2017; 15 (2):23-26.

11. A Primary Mental Health Program in Eastern Province, Saudi Arabia, 2003-2013. Journal of Mental Health in Family Medicine, 2013;10:203-2010.

12. Al-Khathami, A. **Evaluation of Saudi Family Medicine Training Program: The Application of CIPP Evaluation Model,** Medical Teacher Journal; 2012;34 (1):S81-9.

13. Traditional mental health training's effect on primary care physicians in Saudi Arabia. Mental Health Fam Med Journal, 2011 March; 8(1): 3–5.

14. Al-Khathami, A. **Saudi Diploma Program Evaluation: Application of CIPP Model, 2010. [MSc Dissertation Med Education- Cardiff University, UK]**

15. Effect of Mental Health Training Program On Primary-Care Physicians' Skills, Eastern Province, Saudi Arabia, Middle East Journal of Family Medicine , 2007 , 5(4): 22-24

16. Al-Khathami AD. Symptoms analysis of mental illness among Saudi adults attending Primary Care. Neurosciences (Riyadh). 2005 Jan;10(1):73-5.

17. Al-Khathami, A., Can A Short Term Training Course Improve PHC Physicians Attitudes Toward Mental Health Problems? Published in Journal of Family & Community Medicine, 2003 Vol. 10(3): 19-24.

18. Mental Health Training in Primary Care "Impact on Physicians Knowledge" Published in Neuroscience Journal 2003; Vol. 8(2): 447-450.

19. Al-Khathami, A., Prevalence of Mental Illness Among Saudi Adult Primary Care Patients In Central Saudi Arabia, Published in Saudi Med J 2002, Vol. 23(6): 721-724.

20. Al-Khathami, A. Implementation and Evaluation of Educational Program for Primary Care Physicians to Improve their Recognition of Mental Illness in the Eastern Province, Saudi Arabia, 2001. [Dissertation, Fellowship FM, KFU]

CURRENT BOOKS IN PROGRESS

C. A Guide to Medical Teaching and Learning Training of the Trainers (TOT): In the View of the Learner-Centered Learning Model. Partridge Singapore, 2018.

VII-EXPERIENCES

A-Mental Health Care Field:

Leader and trainer of PMHC program since 2002 till now, in same time planer for conducting training courses short and long terms for PHC doctors, and postgraduate residents Diploma and Board certificates. In this program 6 centers in 3 cities. Each center has 3-5 clinics (Family clinic, psychiatry-part time, psychologist, social workers, trained PHC doctors, and nurses). Run regular mental health clinic twice a week since 2002 till now. My postgraduate Fellowship Dissertation subject was in train and evaluate a training course for PHC doctors; Knowledge, Attitude, Practical Skills. Researcher in this field and some papers were published in a scientific journals.

VI - INTERNATIONAL PROFESSIONAL MEMBERSHIP

	ENROLLED DATE
Vice-Chair – Wonca Working Party Group on Mental Health-EMRO	Nov 2016-Now
Affiliated Consultant trainer in Maastricht University	April 2016-Now
Mental Health consultant – Wonca	Nov 2014-Now
Chairman, Trainer Unit Family Medicine – SCFHS	Jun 2014
Representor of WONCA- in WHO Mental Health GAP Forum: Special Focus on Mental Health Action Plan 2013-2020	October 2013, 2015, 2017
Coordinator- Between Wonca Working Party Groups AND Research Group	Jun 2013
Vice-Chair – Wonca Working Party Group on Mental Health	2013-2016
Member – WONCA - Education interest Group	2013
Member – WONCA - Research Interest Group	2013
Member - Mediterranean Regional Mental health Advisory Group (EMERO)	2012 –Now
Member – Local Saudi Family Medicine Board Committee, Saudi Commission for Health Specialties (SCHS)- Eastern Province.	2012 –Now
Member – Local Family Medicine Diploma Committee- (SCHS), Eastern Province.	2010 - Now
Member – Scientific National Committee of Primary Mental Health-M.O.H	2008 – 2010
Member - Postgraduate Family Medicine local committee, Saudi Council for Medical Specialists, King Faisal University - Eastern Province	2005 – 2006
Member – Local Community Mental Health Committee in Eastern Province (M.O.H)	2004-Now
Member - World Organization of Family Doctors (Wonca) Working Party on Mental Health	2004- Now
Editor - Journal of Mental Health in Family Medicine/WONCA, WHO	2004- Now

VII- PROFESSIONAL AFFILIATIONS

1.	Member - Saudi Society of Family & Community Medicine.	2002
2.	Member- American Academy of Family Physicians.	2003
3.	Member- Arab Healthy Water Association (AHWA).	2005
4.	Member - Saudi Psychiatric Association	2006
5.	Member – EMRO Psychiatric Association	2015

VIII- PROFESSIONAL AFFILIATIONS

1.	Member - Saudi Society of Family & Community Medicine.	2002
2.	Member- American Academy of Family Physicians.	2003
3.	Member- Arab Healthy Water Association (AHWA).	2005
4.	Member - Saudi Psychiatric Association	2006
5.	Member – EMRO Psychiatric Association	2015

VI- AS THE TRAINER FOR <u>TOT</u> COURSES

5- Effective Teaching Skills & Portfolio Assessment Course (3days):

Have conducted "Training of the Trainers Courses" over Kingdom

Conducted 12 courses and 238 trainers were trained).

6- Clinical teaching skills & Work-based Assessment Course (2days): 22 trainers in Aseer region. 25 trainer in Arar, 20 in Internal Defense Hosp Dammam, Madina Munora.

Conducted 4 courses

7- Comprehensive TOT Course (5days): 165 trainers were trained in Makkah region, 23 in Riyadh (Shamaisi Hospital), KFH in Riyadh, SPFM-Riyadh-MOH (in 2 periods).

Conducted 5 courses

8- CanMED Roles in Practice and assessment (1day): 185 trainers and resident, Eastern Province-MOH, Asser, Makka, KSU-Riyadh (in 2 periods), PGFM Riyadh (in 2 periods)

Conducted 6 courses

VIII- INTERNATIONAL CONFERENCES & SYMPOSIA – SPEAKER

No.	Title, Place & Date	Duration
1.	Trail of Primary Mental Health Care in Eastern Province, Saudi Arabia, Tripoli, Lebanon, September 2004	3 Days
2.	Implementation & Evaluation of Mental Health Training Program for PHC Physicians, 1st International PHC Conference, Abu Duabi, UAA. Jan. 2006	3 Days
3.	Community Mental Health – Saudi Arabian Pilot, Florence, Italy, Aug 2006	5 Days
4.	The Implementation & The Out-come of Primary and Community Mental Health Program, Saudi Innovation Conference, Newcastle-UK, May 2007	2 days
5	Appling Communication Skills in Patients' Interview in PHC, a Training Course for Family Physicians, Cairo, Egypt, November 2008. a trainer	2 days

6.	November 2008. a trainer Family Health Profile/ Prescribing/ Referral System in Family Practice, Cairo, Egypt, May 2009. a trainer	2 days
7.	International Transcultural Psychiatry Conference, Ranchi, India: 24-25 Sept 2011	2 days
8.	Does intervention training Course improve the PHC physicians' satisfaction and welling to work in PHC centers?. Wonca-2013, Prague, Cz 25-29 Jun, 2013	5 days
9.	Wonca Working Part group on Research meeting and workshops, 24 and 26 Jun 2013, Prague CZ.	2days
10.	Wonca Working Part group on Mental Health meeting, 25 Jun 2013, Prague CZ	1day
11.	International Forum on Innovation in Mental Health, 3-4 October 2013, Lisbon, Portugal	2days
12.	WHO Mental Health Gap Forum: Special Focus on Mental Health-Action Plan 2013-2020, 7th October 2014, Geneva	1day
13.	Learning to work in Integrated Care training professionals for a new service model: Saudi-Portugal Collaboration, 28-30 April 2015, Lila France	3days
14.	Depression and Anxiety among Hypertensive and Diabetic Primary Health Care Patients: Could sleep disturbance be used as a screening tool for Depression and Anxiety?. Wonca-EMRO Conference, Abu-Dubai, 2-4 March 2017	3days

IX- NATIONAL CONFERENCES, SYMPOSIA & WORKSHOPS

Attend a lot of Scientific Activates either a Attendee, Speaker, Organizer, or Trainer

VIII- RESEARCH AND PUBLICATION:

Several researches and contributions were done as illustrated below.

A. Scientific Books

1. **Integrating mental health into primary care:** A global perspective
   World Health Organization and World Organization of Family Doctors (Wonca) 2008, Printed in Singapore. (Contributor)
2. **Companion to Primary Care Mental Health**; 2012,Radcliffe. (Co-Author)

3. Mona Ahmed AlShaikh, Abdullah AlKhathami. Evaluation of Physicians' Communication Skills at Primary Health Care Centers, KSA. INTERNATIONAL JOURNAL OF SCIENTIFIC RESEARCH. 2017; VOLUME-6 (4): 611-618.

4. Abdullah D. AlKhathami, Mohamed A. Alamin, Areej M. Alqahtani, Wafaa Y. Alsaeed, Mohammed A. AlKhathami, Abdulazeez H. Al-Dhafeeri. Depression and Anxiety among Hypertensive and Diabetic Primary Health Care Patients: Could sleep disturbance be used as a screening tool for Depression and Anxiety. Saudi Medical Journal, 2017; Vol. 38 (6): 621-628

5. Rawaf S, Qidwai W, Khoja T, Nanji K, Kurashi N, Alnasir F, Al Shafaee M, Al Shetti M, Bashir M, Saad N, Alkaisi S, Halasa W, Al-Duwaisan H, Al-Ali A, Farahat T, Tarawneh M, Al-Khathami A, Abutiheen A, Iqbal Azam S, Swaka A. New Leadership Model for Family Physicians in the Eastern Mediterranean Region: A Pilot Study Across Selected Countries, 2017. J Fam Med - Volume 4 (2): 1107 page 1-8. www.austinpublishinggroup.com

6. Al-Khathami, A. Leadership in Postgraduate Family Medicine Training Programs: A "Steps-Model" Implementation in Eastern Province-MOH Saudi Arabia. Middle East Journal Of Family Medicine, 2017; 15 (2):23-26.

7. A Primary Mental Health Program in Eastern Province, Saudi Arabia, 2003-2013. Journal of Mental Health in Family Medicine, 2013;10:203-2010.

8. Al-Khathami, A. **Evaluation of Saudi Family Medicine Training Program: The Application of CIPP Evaluation Model**, Medical Teacher Journal; 2012;34 (1):S81-9.

9. Traditional mental health training's effect on primary care physicians in Saudi Arabia. Mental Health Fam Med Journal, 2011 March; 8(1): 3–5.

10. Al-Khathami, A. Saudi Diploma Program Evaluation: Application of CIPP Model, 2010. [MSc Dissertation Med Education- Cardiff University, UK]

11. Effect of Mental Health Training Program On Primary-Care Physicians' Skills, Eastern Province, Saudi Arabia, Middle East Journal of Family Medicine, 2007, 5(4): 22-24

12. Al-Khathami AD. Symptoms analysis of mental illness among Saudi adults attending Primary Care. Neurosciences (Riyadh). 2005 Jan;10(1):73-5.

13. Al-Khathami, A., Can A Short Term Training Course Improve PHC Physicians Attitudes Toward Mental Health Problems? Published in Journal of Family & Community Medicine, 2003 Vol. 10(3): 19-24.

14. Mental Health Training in Primary Care "Impact on Physicians Knowledge" Published in Neuroscience Journal 2003; Vol. 8(2): 447-450.

15. Al-Khathami, A., Prevalence of Mental Illness Among Saudi Adult Primary Care Patients In Central Saudi Arabia, Published in Saudi Med J 2002, Vol. 23(6): 721-724.

16. Al-Khathami, A. Implementation and Evaluation of Educational Program for Primary Care Physicians to Improve their Recognition of Mental Illness in the Eastern Province, Saudi Arabia, 2001. [Dissertation, Fellowship FM, KFU]

http://www.ncbi.nlm.nih.gov/pubmed

C. Current Books in progress
Training of the Trainers (TOT)

VII- EXPERIENCES

A. Mental Health Care Field:

Leader and trainer of PMHC program since 2002 till now, in same time planer for conducting training courses short and long terms for PHC doctors, and postgraduate residents Diploma and Board certificates. In this program 6 centers in 3 cities. Each center has 3-5 clinics (Family clinic, psychiatry-part time, psychologist, social workers, trained PHC doctors, and nurses). Run regular mental health clinic twice a week since 2002 till now. My postgraduate Fellowship Dissertation subject was in train and evaluate a training course for PHC doctors; Knowledge, Attitude, Practical Skills. Researcher in this field and some papers were published in a scientific journals.

B. Postgraduate Family Medicine:

Leader and trainer in Diploma and Board postgraduate Program since 2003 till now.

C. Medical Education:

Have a master degree in Medical Education from Cardiff University-UK, 2010. Design and Conduct several course in this field as Train the Trainers and as subjects in postgraduate programs.

D. Total Quality Management:

A candidate of Diploma program and recognized as Surveyor in CIBAH Primary care (National Standard for the Medical quality accreditation)

Glossary

Application	Ability to implement learned material in concrete situations.
Analysis	Breakdown of the material into its components so that its organizational structure may be better understood.
Assessment Portfolio	An assessment portfolio collects a learner's most typical work or best work on certain themes over a period.
Assessment Processes Purpose	Assessment shifts from assigning grades only to including constructive feedback for the purpose of learning improvement. Integrate assessment with feedback as part of the learning process
Brainstorming	A technique of exploring possible solutions to a problem by generating a wide spectrum of suggestions.
Buzz Groups Technique	The class group (all learners) is divided into small groups of three or four learners to work on a task. There is no need for a group leader.
Direct Observation Of Procedural Skills (DOPS)	Allows an educational supervisor to directly observe a learner undertaking a practical procedure, to make judgements about specific components of the observed procedure, and to grade the learner's performance in carrying out the procedure
Evaluation	Ability to judge, check, or critique the value of material An assessment conducted to determine the effectiveness of the event in meeting the stated learning objectives.
Family Medicine	Family physicians are skilled clinicians who provide comprehensive, continuing care to patients and their families within a relationship of trust. Family physicians apply and integrate medical knowledge, clinical skills and professional attitudes in their provision of care.
Knowledge	Remembering previously learned material.
Canmeds	CanMEDS Physician Competency Framework describes the knowledge, skills and abilities that specialist physicians need for better patient outcomes. The framework is based on the seven roles that all physicians need to have, to be better doctors: Medical Expert, Communicator, Collaborator, Manager, Health Advocate, Scholar, and Professional.
Case-Based Discussion (CBD)	Systematically assesses the learner's performance and explores professional judgment in clinical areas, especially learner thinking (Clinical Reasoning) and problem-solving ability Provides valid, reliable and provide excellent feedback, which is effective and efficient in changing practice. Utilizes professional judgment, which is the ability to make holistic, balanced and justifiable decision in situations of complexity and uncertainty.
Clinical Competence	The degree to which a physician's performance fulfils stated criteria for good clinical practice.

Clinical Teaching	In modern teaching, clinical teaching is a form of social interaction between receptor (clinical teacher) and learners with defined goals around the patients' problems, *not* only around the disease, as in traditional teaching. **It is an opportunity to share information, demonstrate a technique, perform clinical observation, give feedback, and reflect through case discussion.**
Coaching Model	The preceptor acts as an instructor and coach who shows and assists the learners in achieving a set of competencies. The process is collaboration between learner and preceptor. There is a space for the learners to practice certain competencies under supervision. They have a chance to receive feedback on their performance and express their reflections about what they did and what they have learned. This model also called the *competence-based* model and fits junior learners until they master the required clinical competencies.
Collaborator	Work with patients, families, healthcare teams, other health professionals, and communities to achieve optimal patient care.
Communicator	Facilitate the doctor-patient relationship and the dynamic exchanges that occur before, during, and after the medical encounter.
Concept	The underlying meaning, a thought, an abstract idea.
Course/Lesson Plan	It is an important communicational tool for teachers.
Facilitator	Guide the discussion towards achieving the aim of the session, highlight the main points, and help define the learning gap.
Free-Discussion Group Technique	Divide the whole learners' group into small groups, each group consisting of five to nine learners. One of them takes the role of small-group leader and organizes the work within the small group. Each small group selects a presenter(s) to report their task outcome to the whole group.
Health Advocate	Responsibly use their expertise and influence to advance the health and well-being of individual patients, communities, and populations.
LCL Model	Is considered a modern approach in which the learner is actively and effectively engaged in the learning process to master a particular task and create a positive attitude towards it . It is a new approach that uses small-group learning as the learning process. Feedback, reflection, and work-based assessments measure learning achievements.

Learner-Centered Class	Learners participate in leading discussions, and teachers become facilitators. The teacher's role is to facilitate the learners' discussion, allowing learners to learn, use, and explore the learning materials
Learning Portfolio	A learning portfolio includes personal reflective responses to learning experiences.
Learning Responsibility	Responsibility shifts from the instructors to the learners. Instructors guide and motivate learners to become self-directed, lifelong learners.
Manager	They are central to the primary health care team and integral participants in healthcare organizations. They use resources wisely and organize practices which are a resource to their patient population to sustain and improve health, coordinating care within the other members of the health care system.
Method	It is a series of actions using the appropriate teaching technique to acquire knowledge and complete a task.
Modeling Model	The preceptor works as a skilled role model. Learners learn by observing their preceptor's practice. This approach is appropriate for beginners, to make them familiar with their proposed tasks.
Professional	They are committed to the health and well-being of individuals and society through ethical practice, profession-led regulation, and high personal standards of behaviour.
Portfolio	The term "portfolio" is derived from the Latin words *porter* (to carry) and *folium* (leaf, sheet). It is defined as what learner did (Logbook) plus his/her reflection about what were learned.
Power Balance	Instructors share some decision with learners.
Presentation Skills	The presentation is a type of communication in which you transfer your ideas to a group of people in various speaking situations, such as lecture or meeting settings.
Reflective Practitioner Model	The preceptor plays the role of the critical friend or mentor. This step is a based on articulation and exploration of the learners' clinical reasoning through constructive feedback. It is appropriate for senior learners who have already passed through the stages of modeling and coaching. Its process is based on stimulation of self-directed learning through collaboration, and partnership in the learning process between preceptor and learners.
Role Model	Someone who inspires a learner and teaches by example in the course of professional work. Could be a teacher, supervisor or peer.
Role-Play Technique	It is important to repeat the scenario, with learners taking different roles each time. The learner who played the doctor on one occasion, will play the patient on a later occasions, to experience the situation differently. As each play-through of the scenario is finished, constructive feedback should be given.

Royal College Of Physicians And Surgeons Of Canada	A national, private, non-profit organization established in 1929 by a special Act of Parliament to oversee the medical education of specialists in Canada.
Scholar	They demonstrate a lifelong commitment to reflective learning, as well as the creation, dissemination, application and translation of knowledge.
Selection Portfolio	It is a task-based portfolio. The learner provides her or his reflections about events experienced during each training period, e.g., introduction, hospital rotation, and so on.
Self-Efficacy	It is defined as people's beliefs about their capabilities to produce designated levels of performance that exercise influence over events that affect their lives.
Seminar Method	Seminar provides an opportunity for learners to work individually and in a small group to undertake a task based on research and to report back to the whole group for a led discussion.
Small-Group Learning	It is a collection of learners who interact and work together to achieve common learning goals.
Snowballing Technique	It is not dependent upon the learner's preparation for its success. It depends on discussion and criticism of the ideas.
Synthesis	It is a combination of components or elements to form a connected whole.
Technique	It is applied through systematic steps to obtain information and complete a task.
Teacher-Centred Approach	It is known as a *traditional instructional approach*. Teachers are at the centre of classroom activities, including explanations and discussions
Traditional Learning	It focuses on surface learning or memorization. LCL leads to deep learning, connecting current learning to learner experiences and enabling learners to organize their information
Tutorial Method	It is a style of interaction between a teacher and small groups, providing an opportunity for guidance and support.

Bibliography

Ahmad, F. and J. Aziz. Students' Perceptions of the Teachers' Teaching of Literature Communicating and Understanding through the Eyes of the Audience. European Journal of Social Sciences 7 no. 3 (2009):17–39.

J Norcini, V Burch -. AMEE - GUIDE Workplace-based assessment as an educational tool: AMEE Guide. Medical teacher no. 31 (2007).

Amin, Z. and K. Eng.. Basic in Medical Education. Singapore: World Scientific Publishing. 2006.

Anderson, L., D. Krathwohl et al., eds. A Taxonomy for Learning, Teaching, and Assessing: A Revision of Bloom's Taxonomy of Educational Objectives. Boston: Allyn & Bacon. 2001.

Barrows, H. The Tutorial Process. Springfield, IL: Southern Illinois University School of Medicine. 1988.

Baglia, J., E. Foster, J. Dostal, D. Keister, N. Biery, and D. Larson. "Generating Developmentally Appropriate Competency Assessment at a Family Medicine Residency." Family Medicine 43 no. 2 (2011): 90–8.

Blakey. E. and S. Spence. Educational Resource Information Center (U.S. Department of Education), 2008. http://www.education.com/reference/article/Ref_Dev_Metacognition/.

Blumberg. P. Developing Learner-Centered Teaching: A Practical Guide for Faculty. Jossey-Bass. 2009.

Bonwell, C. C. and J. A. Eison. Active Learning: Creating Excitement in the Classroom. ASHE-ERIC Higher Education Report. Washington, DC: George Washington University, 1991.

Branch, William T. and A. Paranjape. 2002. "Feedback and Reflection: Teaching Methods for Clinical Settings." Academic Medicine 77 (2002):1185–8.

Brophy, J. Motivating to Students for Learning. McGraw-Hill, 1998.

College of Family Physicians of Canada. CanMEDS-FM 2017 Working Group. CanMEDS-Family Medicine: A competency framework for family physicians across the continuum, 2017. http://www.cfpc.ca/canmedsfm/

College of Family Physicians of Canada. Defining Competence for the Purposes of Certification by the College of Family Physicians of Canada: The Evaluation Objectives in Family Medicine. Working Group on the Certification Process, 2010.

Crobsy, J. "Learning in Small Groups: AMEE Medical Education Guide No. 8." Medical Teacher 19 (1997):189–202.

Davis, B. Tools for Teaching. 2nd ed. San Francisco: Jossey-Bass, 2009.

Dent. J. and R. Harden. A Practical Guide for Medical Teachers. London: Churchill Livingstone, 2001.

Eken, D. "Through the Eyes of the Learner: Learner Observations of Teaching and Learning." ELT Journal 53 no. 4 (2000): 66–80.

Eraut, M. Developing Professional Knowledge and Competence. London: Falmer, 1994.

Fink, D. L. Creating Significant Learning Experiences: An Integrated Approach to Designing College Courses. San Francisco: Jossey-Bass, 2003.

Fink, D. L. Integrated Course Design. Manhattan, KS: The IDEA Center, 2005. http://ideaedu.org/wp-content/uploads/2014/11/Idea_Paper_42.pdf

Jon O. Neher, Katherine C. Gordon, Barbara Meyer, Nancy Stevens. A Five-Step "Microskills" Model of Clinical Teaching. J Am Board Family no. 5 (1992):419-24.

Harden, R. and Joy Crosby. "AMEE Education Guide No. 20: The Good Teacher Is More than a Lecturer—The Twelve Roles of the Teacher." Medical Teacher 22 no. 4 (2000): 334–347.

Hutchinson, L. "ABC of Learning and Teaching Educational Environment." BMJ 326 (2003): 810–2.

Jaques, D. "ABC of Learning and Teaching in Medicine: Teaching Small Groups." BMJ 326 (2003): 492–4.

Kaufman, D. Applying Educational Theory in Practice: ABC of Learning and Teaching in Medicine. BMJ 326 (2003): 213–216.

Michaelsen, L. K., A. B. Knight, and L. D. Fink. Team-Based Learning: A Transformative Use of Small Groups for Large and Small Classes. Westport, CT: Bergin & Garvey, 2002.

Motivating Students - NDE/NDT Resource Center. https://www.nde-ed.org/TeachingResources/ClassroomTips/Motivating_Students.htm

Motorola University. 1996. "The Learning Pyramid: Creating Mindware for the 21st Century." Corporate University Xchange 2 no 3 (1996).

Muraya, D and G. Kimamo. "Effects of Cooperative Learning Approach on Biology Mean Achievement Scores of Secondary School Students in Machakos District, Kenya." Educational Research and Reviews 6 no. 12 (2011): 726–745.

Newble, D. and R. Cannon. A Handbook for Medical Teachers. 3rd ed. London: Kluwer Academic, 1994.

Norcini, John and Vanessa Burch. 2 1, Foundation for Advancement of International Medical Education and Research, Philadelphia, USA; 2, University of Cape Town, South Africa, Medical Teacher, 29 (2007): 855–871 Shepard 2000

Raaheim, K. et. al. Helping Students to Learn: Teaching, Counselling and Research. Buckingham: Open University Press, 1991.

Reece, I. and S. Walker. Teaching, Training and Learning: A Practical Guide. Oxford: Business Education Publishers, 2006.

Rimanoczy, I. and E. Turner. Action Reflection Learning: Solving Real Business Problems by Connecting Learning with Earning. Mountain View: Davies-Black Publishing, 2008.

Schofield, Susie. Presentation Skills CME, University of Dundee, 2012. http://www.ljlseminars.com/elements.htm.

Spencer, J. and R. Jordan. Learner Centred Approaches in Medical Education. BMJ 318 (1999): 1280–3

Steinert, Y. Twelve Tips for Using Role-Plays in Clinical Teaching. Medical Teacher 15 no. 4 (1993): 283–291.

Tiberius, R. Small Group Teaching: A Trouble-Shooting Guide. Ontario, 1990.

Tuckman, B. original 'Forming-storming-norming-performing' concept; Alan Chapman 2001-2013. http://www.businessballs.com/tuckmanformingstormingnormingperforming.htm review and code.

Weimer, M. Learner-Centered Teaching: Five Key Changes to Practice. Jossey-Bass, 2013.

Index

Printed in the United States
By Bookmasters